OXFORD MEDICAL PUBLICATIONS

Parkinson's Disease and its Management

This book is dedicated to my wife Dr Iris Pearce, who has devoted so much of her time to our patients in the Parkinson's disease clinic; to the treasured memory of my father Dr Wilfred Pearce; and to the future in Simon, David, and Elizabeth.

Parkinson's Disease and its Management

J. M. S. Pearce

Consultant Neurologist, Hull Royal Infirmary

Oxford   New York   Tokyo
OXFORD UNIVERSITY PRESS
1992

Oxford University Press, Walton Street, Oxford OX2 6DP
Oxford New York Toronto
Delhi Bombay Calcutta Madras Karachi
Petaling Jaya Singapore Hong Kong Tokyo
Nairobi Dar es Salaam Cape Town
Melbourne Auckland
and associated companies in
Berlin Ibadan

Oxford is a trade mark of Oxford University Press

Published in the United States
by Oxford University Press, New York

A catalogue record for this book is available from the British Library

Library of Congress Cataloging in Publication Data
Pearce, John, 1936–
Parkinson's disease and its management/J.M.S. Pearce.
Includes bibliographical references.
1. Parkinsonism. I. Title.
[DNLM: 1. Parkinson Disease—diagnosis. 2. Parkinson Disease—
—therapy. WL 359 P359p]
RC382.P36   1992   616.8'33—dc20   92-6176
ISBN 0-19-262177-7 (hbk)

Typeset by Cotswold Typesetting Ltd, Gloucester
Printed in Great Britain by
Bookcraft (Bath) Ltd, Midsomer Norton

Preface

Until 1967 the treatment of Parkinson's disease had been stagnant, but for the modest impact of stereotaxic surgery. The laboratory work of Ehringer, Hornykiewicz, and colleagues in 1960 had drawn attention to the fundamental importance of dopamine as a basal ganglia neurotransmitter. Paradoxically however, they failed to deploy dopamine as a therapeutic agent despite demonstrating its brief clinical efficacy when administered parenterally. It was left to the late George Cotzias in 1967 to show the potential of oral medication with D–L–dopa, and thereby to inaugurate the levodopa ('L–dopa') revolution. The subsequent story of the treatment of the disease has centred on this seminal clinical work.

This short book attempts to provide a practical, concise review of the theory and practice of those factors which bear on correct diagnosis and management. The interested reader will find elsewhere a galaxy of published papers, trial reports, and reviews, and a variety of excellent recent monographs. I have aimed to provide the physician with a full account of the clinical vagaries of the several parkinsonian syndromes and to summarize the relevant knowledge of disordered physiology, pathology, and neurochemistry, so that the clinical dilemmas relating to treatment are intelligible. I have been only too aware of my own deficiencies in the technicalities of modern basic science, and I can only hope that my studies over many years have allowed of a distillate which, if over-simplified, is a basis for the understanding necessary for good medical practice. In the knowledge that modern inter-library reference retrieval is widely available, I have not attempted to provide a comprehensive reference list. I have selected those that I have found most useful, items of historical interest, and up-to-date references for further study on the major topics.

The treatment of Parkinson's disease is both a demanding task and a challenge. If the best results are to be obtained, a multitude of physical and psychological problems have to be confronted. Detailed analysis and scrutiny of the capricious variations in symptoms, disabilities, and reactions to treatments is vital, but time-consuming. Attention to common concurrent illnesses is an essential part of therapy, and sedulous attention to side-effects of drugs, physical therapies, and dietary interactions is vital. Social and physical rehabilitation therapies are not the prerogative of physicians caring for the elderly, but are elements essential to good doctoring in all chronic and disabling diseases, irrespective of age or other artificial categories contrived by administrators and politicians. These aspects are outlined in the text, and certain sections, I hope, may be of service to patients, families, and professional therapists. In treating these patients I have been continually conscious of the pressing need for better welfare services and more humane and dignified domiciliary facilities to replace the presently crude and often impersonal mass provisions of geriatric units and residential homes. Sadly, these are still needed in the more advanced and disabled sufferers; and this need should goad us on to even greater research endeavours to remedy the disorder, or, better, to prevent or modify its assaults on the brain in its earliest stages. Modern studies in these directions are encouraging.

I hope that this small volume will serve trainees and physicians in many disciplines, and ease some of their difficulties in understanding and treating their parkinsonian patients.

Hull   J.M.S.P.
May 1992

Contents

1 Introduction and overview

Accuracy is occasionally impossible; we can only be right in nineteen cases by being wrong in the twentieth. It is well to realize this. But remember that in practice we have to treat that which is only probable as if it were certain. We could not treat two-thirds of our cases properly without doing this.

Sir William Gowers

Since James Parkinson's classic monograph, published in 1817, the disease which bears his name has continued to vex and perplex medical scientists. A vast body of medical literature on the subject has burgeoned in the last 25 years, probably as a result of the singular application of levodopa ('L-dopa') therapy investigated by George Cotzias in 1967 which succeeded the discovery of the fundamental role of dopamine as a central neurotransmitter by Ehringer and Hornykiewicz in 1960.

This small monograph aims to present a concise view of the present state of knowledge, with special emphasis on the management of the varied clinical problems with which patients confront their doctors in surgeries and clinics every day. At the outset, it is encouraging to be able to state that the grim prospects which prevailed thirty years ago have been improved by modern treatments and research—although there is still much to be learned, and much further investigation to be carried out.

This introductory chapter is a *deliberately oversimplified summary* of the salient features, which may prove useful to non-medical professionals and students in search of a brief overview.

Historical note

James Parkinson was the celebrated son of John Parkinson, an apothecary and surgeon to the suburban London village of Shoreditch. James was born on 11 April 1755; he qualified and practised in the fashion of a modern-day General Practioner. Of his six children John, the eldest son, joined him in the practice in Hoxton Square, then a suburb in Shoreditch, London. James was a great social reformer, and also an author, a celebrated biologist and geologist. His essay *On the shaking palsy* was published as a small booklet in 1817. It contains descriptions of six patients he had observed, though it is plain he had not examined them systematically. His clinical prowess is evident in the wealth and subtlety of detail he left us as a legacy in this famous book. It was well received, and it took another forty years before any useful material was added to it. He died in December 1824, four days before Christmas, aged 62.

Working definition

Parkinson's disease is a clinical syndrome characterized by slowness of movement (bradykinesia), rigidity, tremor of the limbs at rest, and disorders of posture. It is due to a degeneration of pigmented nerve-cell systems in the brain.

Epidemiology

The illness may afflict people from all classes of society and all races, and occurs throughout the world. Its rate of incidence increases with aging, but it is not a result of aging itself. Overall, about 1 in 1000 of the population are affected (the prevalence), but this increases to about 1–2 per cent in those in their seventies and eighties. Many elderly people are so mildly affected that in them the disease is easily overlooked. Men and women are equally affected. It is seldom inherited.

Clinical features

The most common early symptom is a rhythmical shaking (tremor) of one or occasionally both hands or arms. Tremor can also affect the legs. It may be accompanied by slowness in movement, loss of skills with tools such as screwdrivers, and difficulty with fine manipulations—fastening buttons, ties, bra fasteners, and shoelaces. The limbs may feel heavy and stiff. Later, relatives may notice a slightly bent, stooped posture, the failure of the arms to swing freely when walking, and a slight lack of facial expression, as if the face is frozen in a mask. The condition can remain stationary for months or years, but usually progresses very slowly.

   It tends to start in the fifties or sixties, but the incidence increases with age, so that between seventy and eighty years of age about one per cent of the population show signs of parkinsonism. The illness is slowly progressive; it may shorten life expectancy, but seldom by any great amount. In the advanced stages, tremor, slowness, and rigidity may affect all four limbs and the trunk; speech may be indistinct and slurred, the limbs and body are bent, and the victim is apt to walk with short, stumbling steps and is prone to fall. Many of these symptoms are controllable by appropriate treatment for many years; the disability is mild, and during this time most patients are capable of normal domestic chores and activities and can usually maintain their normal jobs. Later, as the disease continues, disabilities ensue that ultimately may lead to dependency and a helpless chairbound existence.

Patients sometimes wonder how the diagnosis is made. It is invariably a clinical decision, based on the symptoms, and especially the physical signs, observed during examination. Laboratory tests and X-rays are generally unnecessary, and special tests such as CT scans and MRI scans are unhelpful as a routine; indeed their results are usually normal in Parkinson's disease, though some degree of age-related atrophy is not uncommon. There are a number of other causes of Parkinson-like states (parkinsonism) which have a different pathology, prognosis, and response to treatment. Accurate neurological diagnosis is essential at an early stage; the neurologist will therefore select certain patients for detailed investigation.

Principles of treatment

Treatment is based on the replacement of those chemicals in the brain which are reduced or depleted in Parkinson's disease. The main one is dopamine (derived from the drug levodopa), which diminishes very slowly for many years before any symptoms are apparent. It is estimated that there is a loss of 80 per cent of the dopamine in the critical brain areas before symptoms or signs are evident. Dopamine is widely distributed in the central nervous system, but high concentrations are located in the basal ganglia. Other drugs are also used (Chapter 8).

Physical treatment with physiotherapy, speech therapy, and occupational therapy is valuable at certain stages. The aim throughout is to maintain activity and as near normal a lifestyle as possible. Patients and their families have to be as involved in planning activities, as are the doctors and therapists. Treatment is usually initiated by a neurologist, general physician, or geriatrician in a hospital or private clinic. The general practitioner receives confirmation of his or her diagnosis and advice about treatment, and is invaluable in guiding and in assisting patients at all stages of the illness.

2 History of Parkinson's disease

Before Parkinson's classic *An essay on the shaking palsy* (1817)[1] ancient books recorded many types of paralytic disorders and tremors. None of these fully described the distinctive features of the syndrome which so justly perpetuate Parkinson's name.

His essay referred to the earlier writings of Juncker, who distinguished tremors as either 'Active—sudden affections of the mind, terror, anger' or 'Passive—dependent on debilitating causes such as advanced age, palsy, etc.' Sylvius de la Boe he credited for showing in 1680 the important difference between rest tremor (*tremor coactus*) and action tremor. Parkinson cites Sauvages; 'the tremulous parts leap, and as it were vibrate, even when supported: whilst every other tremor, he observes, ceases, when the voluntary exertion for moving the limb stops ... but returns when we will the limb to move'. He also referred to van Swieten (1749), who had made similar observations about rest tremor. Sauvages had described the *festinant* gait which 'I think cannot be more fitly named than hastening or hurrying Scelotyrbe (*scelotyrbem festinantem, seu festiniam)*', as had Gaubius some ten years earlier (1758).

James Parkinson

Many scholarly writings have been devoted to James Parkinson, his life and work. The reader is referred to McMenemey's essay,[2] Gardner-Thorpe's introduction to the reprint of *The shaking palsy*,[3] and Kenneth Tyler's comprehensive review.[4] Cleevely and Cooper[5] outline his work as a social reformer and geologist, and append an extensive bibliography.

James was born on 11 April 1755, the first child of Mary and John Parkinson. John was an apothecary and surgeon who lived and worked at 1 Hoxton Square in the district of Shoreditch in London. He was Anatomical Warden of the Surgeons' Company, which had replaced the Barbers' Company in 1745 and was succeeded by the Royal College of Surgeons in 1800. In addition to his substantial medical contributions

James was variously described as a radical political pamphleteer (under the pseudonym of 'Old Hubert'), a pacifist, an agitator for parliamentary reform, a member of secret societies, and a campaigner for social welfare. No verified portrait of him exists.

His writing was prolific. His first work was a critical account of medical practice *Observations on Dr Hugh Smith's Philosophy of physic etc.* in 1780. His most famous book was a palaeontological study *Organic remains of a former world*, published in three volumes (1804–11), which ran to three editions. His medical works included: *Some accounts of the effects of lightning; A case of diseased vermiform appendix* (possibly the first account of appendicitis); *Typhoid fever; Hydrophobia; Hints for the improvement of trusses; Gout*; and the *Essay on the shaking palsy*. A crinoid *Apiocrinus parkinsoni*, a gastropod *Rostellaria parkinsoni*, an ammonite *Parkinsonia parkinsoni*, and a stemless palm *Nipa parkinsoni* are other commemorative tokens[5] to this phenomenal and scholarly scientist.

James married Mary Dale in May 1781, and they had six children; two died in infancy, and one son John qualified in Medicine and shared his father's practice. James was afflicted with gout for many years, but is said to have died of a stroke[3] on 21 December 1824. He was baptized, married, and was finally buried in St Leonard's Church.

The shaking palsy

The essay spans only 66 pages and five chapters. A preface offers the reader a conciliatory explanation for a 'publication in which mere conjecture takes the place of experiment', its justification being that the disease of which it treats 'has not yet obtained a place in the classification of the nosologists . . .; whilst the unhappy sufferer has considered it an evil, from the domination of which he had no prospect of escape'. Parkinson stressed the need for 'a continuance of observation of the same case, or at least a correct history of its symptoms, even for several years'. He regretted that 'the disease had escaped particular notice and the task of ascertaining its nature by anatomical investigation'. He hoped pathologists might 'be excited to extend their researches to this malady'.

Parkinson's inquiring mind shines throughout the essay in an array of acute clinical observations and inferences. His descriptions leave one in doubt as to whether he examined his patients in the conventional fashion; but the sharpness of his eye and his qualities as a naturalist are self-evident. As in his quixotic excursions into contemporary politics and the righting of social ills, the essay betrays his deep compassion and humanitarian qualities. Chapter 1 opens with his classic summary:

SHAKING PALSY. (*Paralysis Agitans.*) Involuntary tremulous motion, with lessened muscular power, in parts not in action and even when supported; with a propensity to bend the trunk forward, and to pass from a walking to a running pace: the senses and intellects being uninjured.

The words 'shaking palsy' had been used before, but imprecisely; tremors had been described by Galen, Juncker (tremores paralytoidei), and Cullen. Parkinson noted:

'So slight and nearly imperceptible are the inroads of this malady, and so extremely slow its progress . . . that the patient cannot recall the onset . . . . The first symptoms perceived are, a slight sense of weakness with a proneness to trembling . . . most commonly in one of the hands and arms. . . . in less than twelve months or more, the morbid influence is felt in some other part. After a few more months the patient is found to be less strict than usual in preserving an upright posture.

'As the disease proceeds . . . the hand fails to answer the dictates of the will. Walking becomes a task which cannot be performed without considerable attention. . . . care is necessary to prevent frequent falls. . . . The disease proceeds, difficulties increase: writing can now be hardly at all accomplished; and reading, from the tremulous motion, is accomplished with some difficulty.

Later

the propensity to lean forward becomes invincible, and the patient is forced to step on the toes and fore part of the feet . . . irresistibly impelled to take much quicker and shorter steps, and thereby to adopt unwillingly a running pace. . . . the bowels . . . had all along been torpid, the expulsion of faeces requiring mechanical aid.

Finally

his words are now scarcely intelligible . . . no longer able to feed himself . . . saliva is continually draining from the mouth, mixed with particles of food he is no longer able to clear from the inside of the mouth.

Terminally he describes

sleepy exhaustion, with incontinence and loss of articulation.

Parkinson then provides six beautifully illustrative case histories, of men aged 50, 62, 65, 55, and 72, and of a gentleman whose particulars could not be obtained, ('the lamented subject of which was only seen at a distance'). It is curious that no women were described.

The symptoms—tremor coactus and scelotyrbe festinans, their nature, and the opinions of preceding writers are considered in Chapter 2. Differential diagnosis is considered in Chapter 3. Parkinson emphasized that

this disease does not accord with any which are marked in the systematic arrangements of the nosologists.

He refers to Palsy consequent to compression of the brain, or exhaustion of that organ. He decries the use of the term 'shaking palsy' in convulsive affections, including those of a lady with what we would now call ballistic attacks, and convulsions. Another case cited might be an example of torsion dystonia. He finally describes

> the trembling consequent to the indulgence in the drinking of spirituous liquors and the immoderate employment of tea and coffee—tremor temulentus.

The proximate and remote causes are considered in Chapter 4, along with illustrative cases.

> A diseased state of the medulla spinalis, in that part which is contained in the canal, formed by the superior cervical vertebrae, and extending, as the disease proceeds, to the medulla oblongata

is the proximate cause. Parkinson again expresses his uncertainty, lacking anatomical observations, but postulates injury to the medulla or theca related to the mobility of the cervical spine

> which must render it and the contained parts, liable to injury from sudden distortions.

His cases in this chapter are described for analogy; he realizes they differ substantially from paralysis agitans (a term used by Parkinson in his title-page, but not initiated by Marshall Hall, as is often stated). A man with paralysis and venereal infection, palsies occasioned by injury to the brain, medulla, and upper cord, and Pott's carious disease of the spine are mentioned. This chapter fully portrays the contemporary state of knowledge and the limitations of medical practice and the grave difficulties which beset physicians of the day.

Similarly, Chapter 5, devoted to means of cure, shows us how frustrating attempts at treatment were at that time. Optimism prevails, however:

> there appears to be sufficient reason for hoping that some remedial process may ere long be discovered.

He discusses in turn

> blood taken from the upper part of the neck

and

> ... vesicatories applied to the same part and a purulent discharge obtained by use of the Sabine Liniment.

Later he remarks

> Until we are better informed regarding the nature of this disease, the employment of internal medicines is scarcely warrantable ...'.

This classic and exemplary essay ends by generously extolling the virtues of his colleagues' professional ardour and devotion and

> the benefits bestowed on mankind by the labours of a Morgagni, Hunter, or Baillie'.

Later developments

The essay was well received and cited in Cooke's *Treatise on nervous disease*,[6] in Marshall Hall's celebrated *Lectures on the nervous system*,[7] and by Robert Bentley Todd (of Todd's palsy) in a paper and in his clinical lectures on paralysis.[8] Marshall Hall had access to an autopsy on a 28-year old patient with 'hemi-Parkinsonism' and concluded that the disease was related to a lesion of the corpora quadrigemina; he noted a resemblance to tremor mercurialis. By the mid-1850s the disease was well established, and described in the works of Stokes and Robert Graves[4]; and it is confounded with a description of action tremor in Romberg's Lehrbuch[9]. But little new was added.

Trousseau's fifteenth *Lecture on clinical medicine*[10] was on senile trembling and paralysis agitans. He described rigidity, a sign Parkinson did not pay attention to, and he explained the scelotyrbe festinans: 'as his centre of gravity is thus displaced, he is obliged to run after himself, as it were, so that he keeps trotting and hopping on'. Trousseau also described the progressive slowing of repeated hand opening, the first clear account of bradykinesia. Although James Parkinson had said '*the senses and intellects being uninjured*', Trousseau was aware that 'the intellect . . . gets weakened at last; the patient loses his memory, and his friends notice soon that his mind is not as clear: precocious caducity sets in'. Trousseau was a realist: he had, he said, not cured a single patient with medicaments; pneumonia was the common exitus lethalis, but he was not aware of any autopsy performed in France.

Charcot, Vulpian, and Ordenstein wrote extensively on the Salpêtrière experience which is crystallized[11] in Lecture 5 of Charcot's *Leçons sur les malades du système nerveux* (1877). Their views leaned heavily on Todd's work. Cold, damp, and 'emotions morales vives' were held important. Charcot described the affliction as one of the over-fifties, and classed it as a neurosis, that is, with no proper structural cause. Tremor was the cardinal symptom 'limited at first to one member, then little by little becoming generalized'. Later 'almost pathognomic, the patient closes the fingers on the thumb as though in the act of spinning wool . . . or crumbling bread . . . The movements are slow and seem feeble, although dynamometrical experiments prove that this diminution is not real.' He partly ascribed the weakness to 'the rigidity which prevails in the muscles'.

Charcot recognized 'a tendency to propulsion and retropulsion . . . the individual is unable to stop—being apparently forced to follow a flying centre of gravity'. He referred to the 'peculiar attitude of the body and its members, a fixed look, and immobile features'. He analysed the writing, noting the tremulous fine up-strokes when the down-stroke was firm and relatively normal. Speech was 'slow, jerky and short of phrase ... jolted out as it were, like an inexperienced rider on horseback, when the animal is trotting'. *Parkinson had not commented on the rigidity* of neck, trunk, and extremities; Charcot elucidated these signs and said Parkinson had overlooked them. Bradykinesia was not dependent on rigidity 'dependent neither on the existence of tremors, nor on that of muscular rigidity'. Charcot shrewdly anticipated modern concepts of the movement disorder: a lapse of time between the thought and the act. Terminally 'the mind becomes clouded and memory is lost'. Tremor faded late in the disease, and the final event, as Trousseau had noted, was often pneumonia. His pathological studies added little, but therapeutically he noted the palliative effect of hyoscyamine, the precursor of other belladonna alkaloids.

In *Pathogénie et symptoms de la maladie de Parkinson* in 1895, Brissaud[12] made significant contributions. He remarked on speech as 'murmured, an interminable litany', the voice weakened, without intonation. 'The eyelids were rigid, fashion of trembling ... pupils stenosed and rigid ... At the idea of movement, tremor worsened; with movement itself, tremor ceased.' The synchrony of tremor led him to favour a central origin of the disease. He also observed psychic disorders 'the same repugnance to emit their ideas as to move their limbs'. Paying attention to a crucial paper of Blocq and Marinesco in which hemiplegic parkinsonism resulted from a tuberculoma of the contralateral inferior peduncle, destroying the locus niger, he remarked 'a lesion of the locus niger could very well be the anatomical basis of Parkinson's disease'. At that time nothing was known of the structure or physiology of the substantia nigra, so this was a remarkable and prophetic comment of Brissaud's.

Gowers[13] characteristically surveyed the scene in masterly fashion, reviewing 80 patients of his own. He noted a male preponderance, age of onset 50–60 in half the cases, and a heriditary influence (now disputed) in 15 per cent. Like Charcot he had seldom seen tremor in the face or head. The gait, speech, writing, and the propensity for mental weakness, loss of memory, and a tendency to delusions were clearly enunciated. A mixture of 'arsenic, Indian hemp (cannabis), sometimes combined with opium' was advocated.

Pathology

Parkinson's disease was considered a syndrome of the motor cortex by Gowers and his predecessors, the function and pathophysiology of the basal ganglia being then obscure. Tretiakoff in 1919 examined the brains of 9 parkinsonian patients and noted a variety of degenerative lesions, but pointed out reduced numbers of pigmented cells in the locus niger which he related to disorder of the muscular tone in Parkinson's disease.[14] He also found peculiar concentric inclusions in the cytoplasm of these nigral cells which had been described by F. W. Lewy in 1913. A more complete study of the mesencephalon and its neuropathology formed the basis of a classic paper by Foix and Nicolesco, in 1925,[15] by which time the essential anatomical substrate, which so frustratingly had eluded James Parkinson, was more or less complete.

The pandemic of encephalitis lethargica of von Economo between 1917 and 1926 left in its wake a new variety of disease: post-encephalitic parkinsonism. This was the first of the symptomatic causes of the syndrome recognized, but the clinical features and natural history were substantially different from paralysis agitans. Rare sporadic cases are still described, and its historical importance may be as an indicator of the possibility of slow viral infections of the brain and of their epidemiology and sequelae. Critchley had attempted to separate 'arteriosclerotic parkinsonism' from paralysis agitans. Whether or not a *bona fide* case can be made for a vascular basis for rare examples remains doubtful, though it is still an occasional focus of controversy. A galaxy of striatal Parkinson-like syndromes have been reported. They include progressive supranuclear palsy, multiple-system atropy, and striatonigral and corticobasal degenerations; they are demarcated from idiopathic paralysis agitans.

Recent progress

My undergraduate textbook (Davidson, 3rd edn, 1956) mentions tinct belladonna, tinct stramonium, and hyoscine hydrobromide, and 'newer synthetic preparations Artane, Lysivane and Pipanol'. Great strides have taken place since this time, which are well known. I shall mention them only in outline.

Irving Cooper's serendipitous damage to the anterior choroidal artery whilst ligating an aneurysm in a parkinsonian subject spectacularly controlled contralateral signs; this led to deliberate surgical lesions first in the globus pallidus, then in the ventrolateral nucleus of the thalamus, effected by the ingenious stereotactic devices of the 1950s. Chemo-pallidectomy employed alcohol and other destructive agents; later thermal and cryogenic physical methods were used. Unilateral tremor and rigidity were often abolished with striking benefit; but the central features affecting speech, gait, posture, and balance were either unaffected or sometimes worsened by these procedures.

The levodopa story started in the laboratories of Ehringer and Horny-kiewicz in 1960. The late George Cotzias showed in 1967 that large doses of oral D–L-dopa were clinically highly effective, but I remember the vomiting, fainting, and delay of 2 to 3 months before a stable response was obtained. The pure L-isomer lessened toxicity, and the addition of a dopa-decarboxylase inhibitor was an important step forward. Bob Schwab's discovery of Amantadine and the advent of dopamine agonists followed. But the most significant recent advance has been the experimental model afforded by the (1-methyl-4-phenyl-1,2,3,6-tetrahydropyridine) MPTP contaminants. This was discovered in 1976 when a 23-year old American addict took a shortcut to synthesizing his own pethidine analogue. One by-product was MPTP,[16] which caused severe and pure parkinsonism on the third day, and which responded to L-dopa therapy until his suicide 18 months later. The current excitement concerning fetal nigral transplants awaits the validation of time and future research.

References

1. Parkinson, J. (1817). *An essay on the shaking palsy.* Sherwood, Neely, and Jones, London.
2. McMenemy, W. H. (1955). James Parkinson (1755–1824). A biographical essay. In *James Parkinson,* (ed. M. Critchley). Macmillan, London.
3. Gardner-Thorpe, C. (1987). *James Parkinson.* A. Wheaton and Co., Exeter.
4. Tyler, K. L. (1987). A history of Parkinson's disease. In *Handbook of Parkinson's disease,* (ed. W. C. Keller), pp. 1–34. Marcel Dekker Inc., New York, Basle.
5. Cleevely, R. J. and Cooper, J. (1987). James Parkinson (1755–1824). A significant English 18th century doctor and fossil collector. *Tertiary Research* (Leiden), **8**(4), 133–45.
6. Cooke, R. (1821). History of the method of cure of the various species of palsy. In *A treatise of nervous diseases,* (vol 2, part 1), p. 207. Longman, London.
7. Hall, M. (1841). On the *diseases and derangements of the nervous system.* Baillière, London.
8. Todd, R. B. (1855). *Certain diseases of the brain and other affections of the nervous system.* Lindsay and Blakiston, Philadelphia.
9. Romberg, M. (1840–46). *Lehrbuch der Nervenkrankheiten des Menschen.* A. Duncker, Berlin.
10. Trousseau, A. (1868). Lecture XV: Senile trembling and paralysis

agitans. In *Lectures on clinical medicine delivered at the Hôtel-Dieu, Paris*, (trans, P. V. Bazire). New Sydenham Society, London.

11. Charcot, J. M. (1877). On Paralysis agitans (Lecture V). In *Lectures on the diseases of the nervous system*, (trans. G. Sigerson) pp. 129–56. New Sydenham Society, London.

12. Brissaud, E. (1895). Vingt-deuxieme leçon: pathogénie et symptoms de la maladie de Parkinson. In *Leçons sur les maladies nerveuses (Salpêtrière 1893–1894)*. (ed. H. Merge), pp. 488–501. G. Masson, Paris.

13. Gowers, W. R. (1888). *A manual of diseases of the nervous system*, (2nd edn), pp. 589–607. Churchill, London.

14. Tretiakoff, C. (1919). *Contributions à l'étude de l'anatomie pathologique du locus niger de Soemmering, avec quelques déductions relatives à la pathogénie des troubles de tonus musculaire et de la maladie de Parkinson*. Thesis, Paris.

15. Foix, C. and Nicolesco, J. (1925). *Anatomie cérébrale: les noyaux gris centraux et la région mesencephalo-soux-optique*. Masson, Paris.

16. Langston, W. J. (1985). Mechanism of MPTP toxicity: more answers, more questions. *Trends in Pharmacological Sciences*, **6**, 375–8.

Additional bibliography

Eyles, J. M. (1955). James Parkinson (1755–1824). *Nature* (London), **176**, 580–1.

Jefferson, M. (1973). James Parkinson 1755–1824. *British Medical Journal*, **2**, 601–4.

Knight, D. M. (1974). Chemistry in palaeontology: the work of James Parkinson (1755–1824). *Ambyx*, **21**, 78–85.

Morris, A. D. (1955). James Parkinson. Born April 11, 1755. *Lancet*, **269**, 761–3.

Rowntree, L. G. (1912). James Parkinson. *Bulletin of the Johns Hopkins Hospital*, **23**, 33–45.

3 Aetiology

We are suffering from a plethora of surmise, conjecture and hypothesis. The difficulty is to detach the framework of fact—of absolute undeniable fact—from the embellishments of theorists and reporters.

A. Conan Doyle: *Silver blaze*

Epidemiology

The cause of Parkinson's disease is not known. Clues are available from studies of the distribution of the disease, that is, who is affected, where, and in what circumstances. But these studies are hampered by two factors: incomplete registration in population surveys, and erroneous diagnosis. Misdiagnosis is an important confounding factor. In 15 per cent of cases diagnosed by neurologists in the UK that were subsequently examined pathologically in the 'brain bank', other diagnoses (mostly system atrophies) were demonstrated. In the earlier literature 'arteriosclerotic parkinsonism', post-encephalitic patients, and a number of unrecognized causes of parkinsonism (Chapter 4) confused the epidemiologists' picture and led to erroneous pronouncements. The disorder is common, and the prevalence increases with age (Table 3.1).

Table 3.1 Studies of age-related prevalence per 100 000

Source	Age			
	40–49	50–59	60–69	70–79
Carlisle 1961 (Brewis 1966)	145	162	315	614
Northampton 1982 (Sutcliffe 1985)	15	64	277	702
Aberdeen 1984 (Mutch 1986)	47	78	254	832
Victoria, Australia 1965 (Jenkins 1966)	28	166	297	—

Geographic variation

Perhaps 100 000 patients are affected in the UK at any one time. Men slightly outnumber women in most series, and no race is immune. There is no difference in incidence between social classes. There is quite marked apparent *geographic variation*, with lower prevalence rates in China and Africa (Table 3.2), which may be due to differences in racial

Table 3.2 Geographical distribution*

Place	Prevalence per 100 000
China†	44
Igbo Ora, Nigeria†	58.6
Sardinia, Italy‡	65.6
Northampton, UK§	108
Aberdeen, Scotland‡	164.2
Rochester, Minnesota‡	187
Copiah county, Mississippi†	347

*Data collected from published series, variable criteria, age over 40 in most surveys. Cases ascertained by door-to-door survey †, or from multiple public health records, verified by a physician‡.
§Indicates medical verification may be incomplete.

composition and age-groups ascertained, inaccuracy in surveyors, and in diagnostic criteria. Two USA studies have shown a lower prevalence in black races: 128 and 121 per 100 000 for white men and women versus 30 and 7 per 100 000 for black men and women. Similar data were reported from New Orleans.[1] The intriguing notion that skin melanin might protect the melanin-containing substantia nigra from external toxins has been suggested. Mortality rates are higher in whites than in blacks (1.8 versus 0.4/10 per year) in the USA; but a more recent study shows little difference in age-adjusted prevalence. Differences in mortality data may be due to differing standards of medical care.

Personality types

Despite a number of papers documenting particular personality types and behavioural patterns identifiable before the first physical symptoms appear (Chapter 8), these factors are of secondary importance in what is clearly a physical disease. Aggravation of the illness may however complicate incidental anxiety, emotional or family upsets.

Slow viral infections

As with Alzheimer's disease, attempts to find a linkage with the known slow viral infections of the brain have proved negative.

Age

Although we know it is not due to the normal aging process that affects all our brains, just as it affects other organs, the incidence of Parkinson's disease does rise with age to a peak of about 1 per cent in the 80-year-old. Indeed, a recent Norwegian study shows a prevalence of 5.1 per cent among residents (mean age 81 years, mean duration 9.3 years) in 40 nursing homes.[2] Aging invariably displays its toll in the gradual depletion of brain volume; cortical and white matter atrophy is accompanied by a gradual loss of cell numbers in the nigro-striatum and by reduction in their endogenous dopamine. This occurs in normal aging, to which the parkinsonian subject is not immune. Thus Calne and others have postulated that a combination of genetic and environmental factors may accumulate and accentuate the age-related normal decline in nigral cells and their stores of endogenous dopamine. When a critical level is reached (about 80 per cent dopamine depletion) parkinsonism emerges as a clinical phenomenon. This is an attractive if speculative hypothesis.

Cigarette smoking

Another curious observation is that cigarette smoking has been consistently shown to have a negative correlation with the occurrence of the disease. The mechanism is not known but it has been mooted that nicotine might stimulate endogenous dopamine, or that nicotine or CO might protect the substantia nigra from oxidative radicals.

Environmental toxins

Toxins in the environment have been inculpated since the discovery of MPTP (1-methyl, 4-phenyl-1,2,3,6-tetrahydropyridine)-induced parkinsonism[3]. Historically, there are rare but well-described instances of parkinsonism associated with exposure to mercury, manganese, carbon monoxide, and carbon disulphide. Possible exposure to agricultural pesticides was postulated by Barbeau; but the evidence for disparate incidence in rural and urban areas has varied in different series. Generally, there is an increased incidence in rural dwellers, users of well water, and users of herbicides and pesticides; but some workers have not been able to confirm these findings. Similarly, there is no wholly convincing evidence of clustering in defined geographical areas or in time, and the incidence has not appreciably altered in the last thirty years. (The incidence prior to 1960 is uncertain because the criteria for diagnosis have changed since that time, and because the geriatric population were under-represented and probably not well investigated.) The occurrence of conjugal disease is remarkably low, arguing to some extent against a shared environmental factor. Parkinson's disease is not known to be related to any particular job.

The MPTP story

MPTP causes parkinsonism in both man and primates. It is a chemical contaminant of the illegally made do-it-yourself drugs used by heroin addicts, mainly in California. Young men using these highly dangerous and noxious drugs developed typical parkinsonism within days or weeks. The brains of fatal cases show severe destruction of the substantia nigra, and profound loss of dopamine and other neural transmitters, in a fashion which closely mimics that seen in Parkinson's disease. Their symptoms are controlled by levodopa drugs, which replace the missing dopamine in just the same way as in Parkinson's disease. The brain damage inflicted by MPTP is permanent.

MPTP is not itself a neuronal poison; it is converted by monoamine oxidase B through MPDP to MPP^+. MPP^+ is concentrated in neuromelanin-containing dopaminergic neurons, where it is highly and selectively toxic. MPP^+ is bound to mitochondria, where by free-radical damage it destroys the NADH-linked parts of the Complex-1 which determines the energy metabolic activity of mitochondria, thus depleting ATP and cellular calcium. Cell damage and death result. It is also suggested that MPP^+ can induce the formation of free radicals, causing damage to oxidation pathways, with resulting lipid-membrane peroxidation.

Thus MPTP emerges as a 'protoxin'. To cause cell death it employs the novel mechanism of using the brain's own enzymatic mechanisms

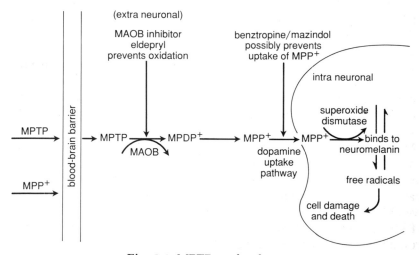

Fig. 3.1 MPTP mode of action.

(MAO-B) within glia to transform it into MPDP and then MPP$^+$. This is an intriguing new concept which raises the question of possible roles for other extrinsic agents, acting as protoxins, to use endogenous mechanisms and thus damage neuronal and other metabolic systems. Genetic, but not necessarily hereditary mechanisms may determine individual susceptibility. Several such metabolic traits may be operative in different subjects.

Toxic radicals

It is known that the breakdown of dopamine by MAO-B generates hydrogen peroxide, which is an oxidative 'stress' on the nigral neurons which are normally protected by enzymes and 'scavengers' of free radicals (Vitamins E and C, reduced glutathione). Recent work has shown that red cell glutathione peroxidase (GP) was lower in 25 late phase patients with severe levodopa fluctuations than in 25 recently diagnosed patients without fluctuations. GP correlated with duration of disease but not with age of patients.[5] This offers one mechanism for susceptibility to extrinsic neurotoxins, since GP normally exerts a protective barrier to toxic free radicals. Aging lessens this endogenous protective mechanism, rendering the neurons more vulnerable to stress from oxidative processes and free radicals. Thus, early exposure in childhood, cumulative exposure to an environmental poison such as MPTP, or a single toxic event may combine with aging and cause nigro-striatal dopaminergic failure.

There are, however, differences between the MPTP model and human disease. The latter always evolves slowly and progressively, whereas MPTP acts as a single noxious insult to the brain, producing symptoms within 2 to 4 days, and evolving over 2 to 6 weeks. Several of the severely affected MPTP patients have, however, shown signs of slow progression after the abrupt onset. Few parkinsonian patients are likely to have been exposed to intravenous MPTP; but of more relevance is the occasional instance of the disease in industrial workers handling the toxin. It is assumed that cutaneous absorption or inhalation may have resulted from cumulative exposure.

MPTP victims show that certain poisons can damage the brain, producing a syndrome similar to that arising spontaneously. And they have provided a most useful model for further research, which is already bearing fruit. Of great interest is the observation that if primates are first given MAO-B inhibitors (e.g. deprenyl or benzotropine) the exposure to MPTP no longer causes the nigral damage. Thus there is a potential for a protective effect of these drugs (cf. selegiline, Chapter 9) if a similar poison is implicated. Researchers are seeking other chemicals which may be present in our environment, but so far none is culpable, and no similar substance has been found in our food or water supplies or in the air we breathe.

Hereditary factors

A positive family history is obtained from probands in between 10 and 50 per cent of cases, allegedly implicating parents and first-degree siblings. Most studies report a positive family history in about 15 per cent of index cases, but much depends on the criteria. There are confusing factors, since examination of all the family members implicated is rarely possible. There is no doubt that many so-called positive family incidences include false positives. These can be due to benign essential tremor; multi-system atrophy (MSA); progressive supranuclear palsy (PSP or Steel–Richardson–Olszewski syndrome); cerebrovascular disease; Alzheimer's disease; diffuse Lewy body disease,[6] and olivopontocerebellar atrophy (OPCA) (see p. 000).

In twin studies Ward, Duvoisin, and colleagues found[7] that the index case had Parkinson's disease in 43 monozygotic pairs, but only two were concordant; in 19 dizygotic pairs only one was concordant. An interesting point in this study was that the prevalence of disease in non-twin siblings (4 of 70 over the age of 60) and parents (6 of 106) was greater than in the co-twins. Marsden's results were similar; 1 concordant of 11 monozygotic pairs, and 1 concordant from 11 dizygotic pairs of twins.[8] (Lack of confirmation by examining the co-twins has been a difficulty which detracts from many of these investigations.) From these data, hereditary factors seem relatively unimportant. However, since there is an enormous number of preclinical cases (with a ratio of preclinical to clinical of 16 to 1 in Forno's pathological studies based on Lewy bodies), there are likely to be 16 preclinical cases for every concordant twin identified in these studies. Re-calculation of the data, if these are included as 'future cases' would change the ratio from 2/43 to 34/43 in Ward's series. This is of course a speculative re-calculation; but the twins studies published do not exclude a genetic factor, and indeed probably underestimate it.

A more demanding but probably worthwhile investigation would be to use positron emission tomography (PET) scanning of 18-fluorodopa in the co-twins and family. This technique has by analogy shown dopaminergic damage in preparkinsonian victims of Guam disease. It might single out individuals destined to develop the disease by demonstrating preclinical but highly significant dopaminergic deficits in the striatum. Affected relatives may share either an increased susceptibility to, or exposure to, some environmental cause which so far we have not identified.

What is the nature of any potential genetic factor? We do not know, but we can consider for comparison the several entities in which a mitochondrial gene is related to neurodegenerative diseases. Mitochondrial encephalo-myopathy with ragged red fibres, Kearns–Sayre syndrome, and Leber's optic atrophy are well-known examples. They are generated by mutations in the mitochondrial genome. Mitochondrial Complex-1 is a major part of the system, and has been shown to be depleted in the substantia nigra and in platelets in parkinsonian subjects when compared to controls. The affinity of MPP$^+$ for the Mitochondrial Complex-1 is a fascinating observation which may be relevant if this site is genetically enfeebled, and thereby vulnerable. Golbe has pointed out that a weakness of this hypothesis is that the mitochondrial genome is absent from sperm, so that paternal transmission by this method would be impossible.[9] Meanwhile researchers have started to locate 'susceptibility gene loci', and we hope that sequencing and transcription may follow. This might permit preclinical detection and prophylaxis, in due course.

Neuropathology

A simple review of the neuropathology explains the morphological damage seen in the disease, and poses unanswered questions as to how this comes about. Apart from age-related atrophy of cortical gyri and variable enlargement of the ventricles, the parkinsonian brain is remarkably normal on gross inspection, with the notable exception of pallor of the normally dark substantia nigra. Highly characteristic, but non-diagnostic, Lewy bodies and glial foci are the major features on microscopic examination. They are found most strikingly in the compact zone of the substantia nigra and in the similarly pigmented (noradrenergic) locus coeruleus of the midbrain. Lewy bodies are also seen in autonomic ganglia, the substantia innominata, the amygdala, the hypothalamus, and the dorsal motor nucleus of the vagus; they may be seen throughout the cortex in smaller numbers. Those groups of nerve cells carrying neuromelanin pigment are the main sites where Lewy bodies are found, and always show signs of degeneration. Neuromelanin may be the result of breakdown of intracellular catecholamines, including dopamine; but whether it protects the cell or is itself toxic when it accumulates is uncertain. It is of interest that it is preserved in albinos.

Another focus of interest is the neurotrophin family—nerve growth

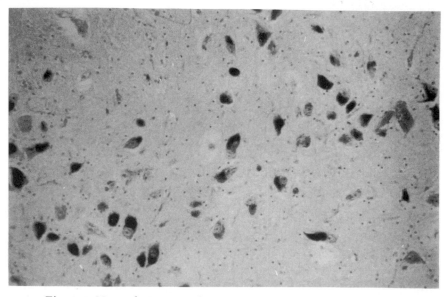

Fig. 3.2 Normal pigmented nerve cells of the substantial nigra.

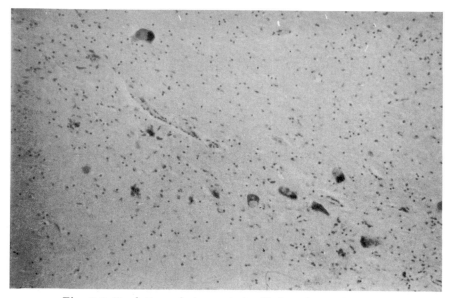

Fig. 3.3 Depletion of pigmented cells in substantia nigra.

factor (NGF), neurotrophin-3, and brain-derived neurotrophic factor (BDNF). NGF stimulates the growth of sensory and sympathetic neurons, but not dopaminergic neurons; by contrast BDNF protects against the loss of dopaminergic cells containing tyrosine hydroxylase, and reduces the neurotoxic effect of MPP$^+$ *in vitro*.[10] It has been shown to be technically feasible to infuse NGF to support adrenal autografts; but it is too early to assess either the aetiological role or the therapeutic importance (if any) of neurotrophins in Parkinson's disease.

Lewy bodies

Lewy bodies are neuronal inclusions present in practically every case. They are pink acidophilic blobs, and show a central core with a peripheral halo. They are multiple, sited in the cytoplasm of neurons. Under electron microscopy they show radiating filaments resembling Van Gogh's sunflowers. They are composed of proteinaceous degenerating neurofilaments.

They are also seen in 5 to 10 per cent of normal brains of those aged over 60, and in 10 per cent of cases of Alzheimer's disease. Their presence therefore is not diagnostic. Their numbers do not correlate with the duration or the severity of the disease.

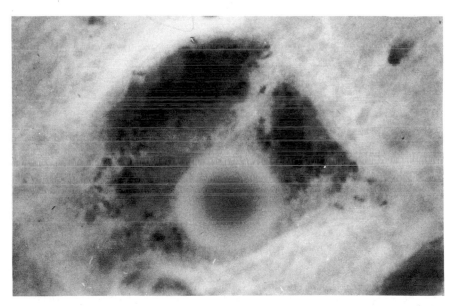

Fig. 3.4 Lewy bodies showing concentric hyaline inclusions in the cytoplasm and halo.

Lewy bodies can be found in the cortex, and there they are related to the incidence of dementia. In **cortical Lewy-body disease** dementia typically precedes parkinsonian features and may represent an entity different from the typical brainstem Lewy-body pathology[11] which characterizes classic Parkinson's disease. By means of modern ubiquitin staining, a dramatic picture of the number and widespread distribution of degenerating neurons can be shown.

Biochemistry

Dopamine

This is not the place for a detailed account of the many biochemical aberrations in Parkinson's disease. It is important, however, to understand the basic problems if drug treatment is to be logical. Destruction of the mesolimbic dopaminergic system is the hallmark of the disease (Fig. 3.5). We have mentioned that 80 per cent of dopamine is lost from the nigrostriatal neurons before clinical signs emerge. Similarly, the specific synthesizing enzyme tyrosine hydroxylase and the less specific dopa-decarboxylase are both reduced in the putamen, caudate, and nigra. Tyrosine is hydroxylated to levodopa which in turn is decarboxylated to dopamine (Fig. 3.6). Thus the use of the peripheral dopa decarboxylase inhibitors, carbidopa and benserazide, reduces peripheral side-effects but potentiates central dopaminergic activity. Dopamine is then metabolized by two routes; by monoamine oxidase

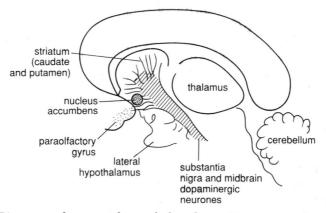

Fig. 3.5 Diagram of meso-telencephalic dopamine system (parasaggittal plane). [Modifed from Hornykiewicz, O. (1982). *Neurology 2. Movement disorders*, (ed. C. D. Marsden and S. Fahn), Ch. 4, p. 43. Butterworth.]

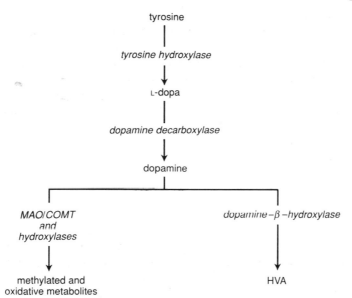

tyrosine

tyrosine hydroxylase

L-dopa

dopamine decarboxylase

dopamine

| MAO/COMT and hydroxylases | dopamine–β–hydroxylase |

| methylated and oxidative metabolites | HVA |

Fig. 3.6 Metabolism of tyrosine and dopamine.

catechol-O-methyltransferase to methylated and oxidative metabolites, and also by the enzyme dopamine-β-hydroxylase to noradrenalin and homovanillic acid (present in CSF).

Depletion of dopamine is most evident in the putamen, which projects on to the ventrolateral nuclei of the pars compacta of the substantia nigra. Striatal dopamine deficiency is the principal cause of parkinsonian symptoms and signs, irrespective of the aetiological type. The depletion of dopamine parallels the severity of neuronal damage. There is also an ascending dopaminergic system in the tegmentum of the midbrain which projects upwards to the cortex and limbic areas in humans (Fig. 3.5), though cortical dopamine levels are normally only about 1/500 of those in the nigrostriatum.

Other neurotransmitters

Many other neurotransmitters are impaired in Parkinson's disease (see also Chapter 6). Cell bodies in the locus coeruleus, which is noradrenergic, the Meynert's nucleus, which is cholinergic, and the long ascending fibres from the serotonergic reticular formation are all depleted at both structural and biochemical levels. Amongst the many neuronal markers depleted (Chapter 6), there are five neuropeptides of interest: met-enkephalin, leu-enkephalin, somatostatin, substance P, and cholecystokinin. There is unfortunately little basis on which we can correlate these findings with clinical symptomatology, though the fairly selective depletion of somatostatin in the cortex may relate to the dementia found in about 10 to 20 per cent of patients.[12] Cholinergic depletion has been thought to play some part in memory function. Noradrenalin deficiency may contribute to akinesia and freezing, but more importantly may related to the common depressive illness seen both before and after the onset of the parkinsonian illness. The inhibitory GABA system may also be depleted, as is shown by reduced glutamic acid decarboxylase (GAD) levels; but measurements are influenced by agonal changes and are therefore not reliable.

Biochemical conclusion

From the complex *mélange*, the principal abnormality remains that of severe and progressive striatal dopamine depletion. It is known that normal nigrostriatal function utilizes dopamine to effect the fine tuning of motor control of the whole body. Dopamine deficiency leads therefore to a major part, if not the whole, of the mechanism of breakdown of the motor system.

Many physiological abnormalities result from dopamine depletion; many can be seen and measured at the bedside as clinical signs which permit attempts at understanding the symptoms and disabilities incurred by patients. They are also valuable methods of observing the progression of the illness, and the effects of treatment.

References

1. Paddison, R. M. and Griffith, R. P. (1974). Occurrence of Parkinson's disease in black patients at Charity Hospital in New Orleans. *Neurology*, **24**, 688–91.
2. Larsen, J. P. (1991). Parkinson's disease as community health problem: study in Norwegian nursing homes. *British Medical Journal*, **303**, 741–3.
3. Langston, J. W., Ballard, P., Tetrud, J. W. *et al.* (1983). Chronic parkinsonism in humans due to a product of meperidine-analog synthesis. *Science*, **219**, 970–80.
4. Tanner, C. M. and Langston, J. W. (1990). Do environmental toxins cause Parkinson's disease? A critical review. *Neurology*, **40**, (Suppl. 3), 17–30.
5. Johannsen, P., Velander, G., Mai, J., Thorling, E. B., and Dupont, E. (1991). Glutathione peroxidase in early and advanced Parkinson's

disease. *Journal of Neurology, Neurosurgery, and Psychiatry*, **54**, 679–82.

6. Joachim. (1988). Lewy body Parkinson's disease. *Annals of Neurology*, **24**, 50–6.

7. Ward, C. D., Duvoisin, R. C., Ince, S. E. *et al.* (1983). Parkinson's disease in 65 pairs of twins and in a set of quadruplets. *Neurology*, **33**, 815–24.

8. Marsden, C. D. (1987). Parkinson's disease in twins. *Journal of Neurology, Neurosurgery, and Psychiatry*, **50**, 105–6.

9. Golbe, L. I. (1990). The genetics of Parkinson's disease: reconsideration. *Neurology*, **40** (Suppl. 3), 7–14.

10. Hyman, C., Hofer, M., Barde, Y.-A. *et al.* (1991). BDNF is a neurotrophic factor for dopaminergic neurons of the substantia nigra. *Nature* (London) **350**, 230–2.

11. Forno, L. S. (1987). The Lewy body in Parkinson's disease. In *Advances in Neurology*, Vol. 45, (ed. M. D. Yahr and K. J. Bergmann), pp. 35–43. Raven Press, New York.

12. Agid, Y., Ruberg, M., Raisman, R., *et al.* (1990). The biochemistry of Parkinson's disease. In *Parkinson's disease*, (ed. G. Stern), pp. 99–126. Chapman and Hall, London.

4 Clinical features of Parkinson's disease

An outline of the main clinical features is given in Chapter 1. Here they are described in more detail, together with some physiological data which explain many of the apparent quirks of behaviour and movement which determine patients' disabilities and the dilemmas posed by treatment. Parkinson's observations in his *Essay* are quoted at the head of the relevant sections.

Symptoms vary a great deal. Some patients, for example, never develop a tremor—the so called rigid-akinetic syndrome; most of these patients have symptomatic parkinsonism, and demand investigation and careful follow-up.

All symptoms fluctuate, even in the untreated state. Sleep confers great benefit on some sufferers, and it is therefore not surprising that even in well-established levodopa-treated disease, some patients are energetic and independent on rising in the mornings, often 12 hours or more after their last dose of medication. Others at the same stage have marked early-morning akinesia and inertia, which is only relieved after their first dose of drugs takes effect.

Psychological factors are important; but responses to stress, depression, and emotional crises are variable, although they generally worsen symptoms temporarily, if not affecting the actual natural history of the malady.

Table 4.1 lists the more common physical signs:

Tremor

The first symptoms perceived are, a slight sense of weakness with a proneness to trembling ... most commonly in one of the hands and arms ... in less than twelve months or more, the morbid influence is felt in some other part.

The commonest early symptom, found in about 75 per cent of patients, is shaking of one hand or, less commonly, both. It is a rhythmical, slow **rest tremor**, at 4–6 Hz, reduced or abolished when the limb is in action. 'Pill-rolling' is the classic description of the early signs of tremor between

Table 4.1 Some common physical signs

- akinesia, hypokinesia, and bradykinesia, for example poor finger dexterity, micrographia; slow starting movements; poverty of spontaneous actions;
- lead pipe and cogwheel rigidity;
- slow rhythmic 'pill-rolling' tremor';
- lack of normal automatic movements, for example, lack of fidgeting, leg crossing and uncrossing; unnatural stillness;
- flexed 'simian' posture of trunk and limbs;
- steps are short and shuffling, feet appear frozen to the ground;
- face masking: lack of expression;
- infrequent blinking, eyes tend to stare;
- dribbling, reduced swallowing of saliva;
- voice is quiet, hoarse (dysphonia);
- speech dysarthric;
- glabella tap sign positive.

the thumb and the flexed index finger; but the process often involves the whole hand and wrist, and when it is severe the whole limb may shake and transmit its aberrant motion to the trunk. Resting tremor is a compound tremor, never simply in one plane, but commonly varying, with both rotational pronator–supinator and flexor–extensor movements.

Some patients also have a **postural tremor**, which is faster, at 6–8 Hz. It is uncertain whether this is exaggerated 'physiological tremor' or a separate pathophysiological release phenomenon. Postural tremor may be the cause of the ratchet-like sensation felt on passive movement of a limb, which is well known as the 'passive cogwheel' phenomenon.

Rest tremor usually vanishes in sleep. Movement diminishes it, but it recurs a few seconds later. Tremor is intermittent at first, more prominent when a visitor or doctor causes temporary excitement, and always worse during periods of apprehension or anxiety. It is often increased when the patient arises from a chair and starts to walk. Movement of one limb, for example, clenching and unclenching the fist will activate tremor in the opposite limb, a useful bedside test for latent tremor.

Electromyography (EMG) shows alternating contraction of agonist and antagonist muscles. Lesions of the substantia nigra do not cause tremor in primates, but experimental lesions in the ventral midbrain tegmentum do. Lesions to the cerebellar outflow to the thalamus and red nucleus do not cause tremor, but any dopamine-depleting drug applied to lesioned animals produces typical rest tumour. Thus the basis is probably a combination of reduction in nigrostriatal dopamine and damage to the efferent cerebellar pathways.

Lesions of the pyramidal tracts do not inhibit tremor, but for tremor to be present an intact cortex and ventrolateral nuclei of the thalamus are necessary. It is thought that in man there is a natural intermittent *generator* of rhythmic bursts of neuronal activity arising in the thalamus which interconnects with the cortex. Stereotaxic operations have successfully and often dramatically abolished tremor. Though it has been superseded by drug-treatment elsewhere, Japanese workers still carry out this operation for intractable tremor, the site of choice being the nucleus ventralis intermedius (Vim), which corresponds to the results of experiments in monkeys.

The putative central oscillator is modulated by an afferent loop deriving from proprioceptors in muscle spindles and by projections from the spinal cord. There is much uncertain terrain in the study of tremor. We do not yet understand the precise location and interactions of the generator producing tremor via the motor cortex. We also have little evidence of cerebellar efferent, red nucleus, or thalamic pathology in man; yet this seems a prerequisite for rest tremor in other primates.

Rigidity

Curiously, *Parkinson did not specifically mention rigidity in his essay.* Charcot pointed this out in 1868: 'overlooked by Parkinson as well as his successors'. Rigidity describes the clinical phenomenon of increased resistance to passive movement, perceived by the examiner more or less equally in agonist and antagonist muscles. It is detectable at an early stage in almost all subjects (for example, 97 per cent at first examination).[1] It is best described as 'lead-pipe', with its even, plastic sense of resistance. It is more obvious in flexor than extensor muscles, and this is in part responsible for the generalized flexed attitude. The 'cogwheel' phenomenon is present in many subjects, and probably reflects the superimposition of postural tremor (6–8 Hz) on 'lead-pipe' resistance.

Rigidity is first detectable in the posterior neck muscles and shoulders. When the patient lies on his back on the couch, his head may remain flexed forward for many minutes, leaving a space betweeen it and the cushion—the 'psychic pillow'. Truncal rigidity is easily overlooked or mistaken for postural abnormality. If the patient's shoulders are swung from behind, the rigid arm(s) fail to swing passively (Wilson's sign). The legs are much less rigid than the arms in most patients. Rigidity may sometimes be found in one arm whilst tremor is more noticeable in the other, showing that the two phenomena are independent. Its incidence varies, being worse during arousal and during exertion.

Rigidity contributes to the immobile mask-like *facies*, as does hypokinesia. It is also found in association with dystonic posture in the fingers of the parkinsonian hand in advanced illness, with its flexion at metacarpo–phalangeal joints and the extended interphalangeal joints, with the swan-like tapering of the fingers and ulnar deviation at the wrist. Rigidity may also be associated with the pain felt diffusely in the back and shoulders, and is probably related to the common 'frozen shoulders' with adhesive capsulitis which may *precede* or occur at any time during the illness. To the patient it means stiffness and a sense of effort required to move the limb, which may feel heavy and weak, though loss of strength and power is not a feature of Parkinson's disease. Levodopa, anti-cholinergic drugs, and also stereotactic surgery on thalamic and pallidal nuclei may each reduce rigidity, hinting at the complexity of the anatomical and neurotransmitter systems at fault.

Physiologically, rigidity is reduced by dorsal root section, showing that afferent input from joint and muscle proprioceptors is a factor. Muscle-spindle activity is normal if the subject is capable of relaxing his muscles, but usually there is hyperactivity, showing increased fusimotor activity in the gamma efferent pathways. Spinal reflexes, tendon reflexes, H-reflexes, antidromic F-reflexes, and tonic vibration are probably normal, though experimentation involves complex techniques and more work is to be done. Long-latency reflexes arise when muscles are briskly stretched and a late response is evoked dependent on longer loops to the sensorimotor cortex or on slower conducting secondary spindle afferents in the cord. Whatever their mechanism, they are testable, and have been found to be exaggerated in Parkinson's disease,[2] as is the excitability of anterior horn cells. Correlation with rigidity is not constant and other factors such as the increased tonic response to sustained static stretch may be of more fundamental importance. For an excellent review, see Marsden 1990.[3]

Slowness of movement

As the disease proceeds ... the hand fails to answer the dictates of the will. Walking becomes a task which cannot be performed without considerable attention. ... care is necessary to prevent frequent falls. ... The disease proceeds, difficulties increase: writing can now be hardly at all accomplished; and reading, from the tremulous motion, is accomplished with some difficulty.

Impaired movement, a seminal feature, is present in almost every case; it is observable in many ways. The man noticed in front of you in the theatre, sitting so still that you wonder if he is asleep—or worse—betrays the striking lack of spontaneous and automatic movement which characterizes the illness. Lighting a cigarette (to protect against further ravages of the illness!) is carried out as if in slow motion (see p. 31). The start of each movement is perceptibly delayed. The smallest possible number of muscle groups are activated, so that the associated movements of shoulder and elbow, which combine normally to produce an elegant smooth and co-ordinated sequence, are missing. The same patterns are apparent when he walks, or arises, or sits down in a chair. Hypokinesia is manifest in infrequent blinking, in the frozen mask-like slow movements of facial expression, in the tongue, and sometimes in speech—although rapid, lalling, monotonous speech, with both dysarthria and dysphonia is more typical of advanced cases.

Axial apraxia

Laboured motion of the axial muscles troubles patients who try to turn over in bed, rise from a chair, or get up from the floor; these difficulties are compounded by a more fundamental defect of the cerebral organization of movement—'**axial apraxia**'—in which it is clear that the choice of movements is inappropriate for the task in hand. This is seen in the patient attempting to rise from a chair who insists on leaning backwards with legs extended, so that it is impossible for him to swing his centre of gravity forward and achieve purchase on his forefeet.[4] Dexterity is affected, with progressively diminishing size of written letters—**micrographia**. There are great difficulties in fine movements, for example, fastening buttons and zips, or tying shoelaces. The gait is halting, steps are short, the arms fail to swing naturally. The slowness is nearly always bilateral, though it may predominate on one side; this gives the lie to the foolish term 'hemiparkinsonism'.

Clinical tests

Clinical tests are useful and include samples of writing, drawing spirals, sinusoidal lines, measured speeds of tapping, and counting the number of insertions of pegs into a pegboard in one minute. Step length and walking speed over a set distance can all be measured for assessment and future reference (see also Chapter 8).

Physiology of akinesia

The physiological basis of akinesia is not clear, though it is a fundamental *sine qua non* of the disorder. It is not improved by stereotactic operations which may benefit tremor and rigidity. It is improved by levodopa drugs, which in the early stages may virtually abolish this symptom. A failure to select and programme the right agonist muscles in advance of rapid and precise movement appears to be a fundamental defect. Further, studies measuring the separate or simultaneous execution of simple movements (for example, flexing the elbow and squeezing a strain gauge) show that both components are slow, that there is an abnormal delay in switching from one movement to the other, and that there is difficulty in executing the actions simultaneously. Current speculations propose a defect in the basal ganglia in directing the sensorimotor cortex to select and organize the motor programmes encoded by past experience.[5]

The essential features are:

1. Impaired storage or delivery of stored patterns of planned skilled or complex movements in the brain.
2. Difficulty in doing two things at once.
3. Impaired ability to carry out sequences involved in motor tasks.
4. Abnormal postures and 'apraxia' of limbs, and especially of axial muscles.
5. Impaired righting reflexes—victims cannot save themselves from a fall. Poor awareness of their centre of gravity and body position (more agnosic than apraxic?).
6. Rigidity of trunk and limbs, representing tonic stretch reflexes; these rigidities contribute to bradykinesia, but are not the primary source.
7. Akinesia—inability to initiate movement; bradykinesia—slow execution of movement; hypokinesia—reduction of spontaneous and automatic movements and the range of amplitude of motor actions. These are the cardinal 'negative symptoms' of the disease.

Disorders of posture

After a few more months the patient is found to be less strict than usual in preserving an upright posture. ... the propensity to lean forward becomes invincible, and the patient is forced to step on the toes and fore part of the feet ... irresistibly impelled to take much quicker and shorter steps, and thereby to adopt unwillingly a running pace.

Here we must consider the dystonic flexed postures of the neck, trunk, and limbs which develop. The arms are held close to the sides, elbows and wrists slightly bent; the legs too may be flexed at the hips and knees. The parkinsonian hand described above (and on p. 29) and the plantar-flexed inverted foot are also evidence of the dystonia. Failure of postural reflexes explain some of the most refractory symptoms. Impaired righting reflexes cause patients to fall after tripping. The freezing to the ground associated with akinesia is due in part to a demonstrated failure of forward and side-to-side sway at the trunk and hips, which is necessary to initiate the next step.

Impoverished awareness of the centre of gravity is part of the defective motor programme held in the cortex and basal nuclei. The characteristic forced running—propulsion, and also retropulsion—seems to be due to a lack of inhibitory impulses, possibly influenced by inappropriate responses to vestibular and proprioceptive cues. Akinesia and some element of rigidity are additional factors; but there remains much of the uniquely disordered gait, stance, and turning which remains enigmatic.

As the ailment progresses steps becomes shorter and slower, the arms fail to swing automatically during walking, the neck and trunk are increasingly bent, and the gait becomes more unstable, punctuated by frequent trips, falls, and injuries.

Disordered eye movement is present in many patients.[6] Slight impairment of vertical up-gaze and convergence are clinically evident. Delayed reaction times are present for both visually-guided random and non-random saccades. There is evidence that these defects are due to a deficiency of dopamine. Quantitative electro-oculography shows that smooth pursuit movement velocity is also reduced. Opticokinetic reflex responses show a reduced velocity, probably a reflection of defective reflex pursuit movement. Vestibulo–ocular reflexes do not differ from those found in control subjects.[6] Impaired ocular saccades in following a remembered target show dysmetria and a multi-step pattern, probably reflecting impaired function between the basal ganglia and the superior colliculus, or between basal ganglia and the cortical projections destined for the superior colliculus.

Smooth muscle disorder

... the bowels which had all along been torpid, the expulsion of faeces requiring mechanical aid.

Constipation

Constipation is almost invariable and is attributed to 'bradykinesia' of intestinal peristalsis. It causes a great deal of obsessional concern to patients, but seldom causes intestinal obstruction, though spurious diarrhoea is frequent in the advanced disease and in the elderly. Liberal supplies of added dietary bran and fibre are preferable to purgative abuse, which is, not surprisingly, frequently encountered.

Hoarseness and dysphagia

Hoarseness may be due to impaired function of laryngeal muscles and the vocal cords. **Dysphagia** may occur, generally late in the illness;

abnormal oesophageal contraction waves can be demonstrated on cine-barium studies.

To the physician these problems pose difficulties because a coincidental neoplasm may develop, also causing altered bowel habit, hoarseness, or dysphagia. Each patient requires careful assessment to exclude such non-parkinsonian complications. Weight loss is also very frequently found in Parkinson's disease (Schwab), and may lead to an unrevealing quest for an occult neoplasm.

Bladder problems

Bladder problems are common and result from ineffective hyper-reflexic detrusor contractions (75 per cent of patients) and external sphincter dysfunction (17 per cent) shown on urodynamic studies.[7] Voluntary sphincter control is indicated by the patient producing on request contractions of the perineal muscles; this can be demonstrated clinically or measured by perineal electromyography.[7] When a subject is unable to suppress detrusor contraction when the bladder is filling during a urodynamic study, detrusor hyper-reflexia is present. Any tendency to prostatism is aggravated when the detrusor power is insufficient to overcome bladder-outlet obstruction. Urge incontinence, frequency, and a poor stream are the common symptoms; incontinence occurs in 5–10 per cent of male patients. Prostatectomies are performed when there is a definite mechanical obstruction due to hyper-trophy, but the results are less favourable than in non-parkinsonian patients. Post-prostatectomy incontinence occurs in 20 per cent of parkinsonian patients who have poor or absent voluntary sphincter control before the operation. In the continent patient, the risk of incontinence after the operation is about 4 per cent, compared to 1 per cent in the non-parkinsonian population.

Sexual disorders

Over half of all patients have sexual disorders, particularly infrequency and avoidance of intercourse. Lack of orgasm is common in females; dissatisfaction, premature ejaculation, and impotence in males. Poor communication and lack of sensuality are common to both sexes. Possible autonomic dysfunction occurs in over 40 per cent of these patients but, as with depression and levodopa treatment, does not correlate closely to the occurrence of sexual problems. The issue is strikingly worse when the affected patient is male.[8]

Other features

Hyposmia. Many parkinsonian patients have diminished or absent sense of smell.[9] Odour-identification test scores have shown that 90 per cent of patients fall below the normal range for detecting different smells, and 75 per cent had impaired sensitivity to actual threshold.[9] These deficits appear early and appear to be unrelated to disease duration. Their cause is obscure, and the finding is non-specific in view of the high incidence of varying degrees of hyposmia in the population.

Seborrhoea. This is a well known finding, featuring (probably unnecessarily) in the Webster scoring scale. It was more frequent in post-encephalitic than in idiopathic disease, but still occurs in some patients with neuroleptic-induced parkinsonism, and in occasional cases of pseudo-parkinsonism associated with vascular disease. Curiously, an oily, acne-studded skin is observed in MPTP disease, even before the motor signs declare themselves.

Radiological investigations

Computed tomography (CT) is normal in many patients. With advancing age some degree of central white matter atrophy causing ventricular dilatation, and gyral atrophy with enlarged sulci, are visible in a high proportion of non-parkinsonian patients. Thus mild degrees of CT-demonstrated atrophy are unremarkable. Attempts to show a greater degree of atrophy or atrophy appearing at an earlier age have shown inconsistent findings in parkinsonian subjects. Such atrophy, when shown, shows no convincing correlation with the cognitive decline present in some of these patients.[10]

MRI studies in 30 patients and 10 matched controls have shown that the surface area of the brain at the level of the foramen of Monro and ventricular measurements did not differ significantly between patients with dementia, patients without dementia, and controls.[11] Some workers have claimed to show reduced dimensions and altered signal brightness of the substantia nigra; this may depend on the imaging techniques, and the observation requires confirmation.

Natural history

Finally 'his words are now scarcely intelligible . . . no longer able to feed himself . . . saliva is continually draining from the mouth, mixed with particles of food he is no longer able to clear from the inside of the mouth'. Terminally he describes 'sleepy exhaustion with incontinence and loss of articulation'.

The mean age of onset is not easy to determine because of changes in the age structure of the population in the last few decades which have resulted in far more patients becoming afflicted in their seventh and eighth decades. The mean age is now between 60 and 65 years. Progression is gradual and inexorable in most patients. Kinnier Wilson remarked on its 'unremitting course and intractable nature'. However, periods of arrested progression, when the symptoms appear to be static, are not uncommon, particularly in the first three or four years of onset. A significant minority, perhaps 10–15 per cent, appear to remain static without clinical deterioration for twenty years or more; they were regarded by Schwab as a 'benign group', and doubtless their fundamental nigrostriatal dysfunction is of different pathogenesis from the classic type of the disease. Five stages have been arbitrarily assigned by Hoehn and Yahr[12] (Table 4.2).

Table 4.2 Stages of disease (Hoehn and Yahr, 1967)

I.	duration	3*	unilateral disease only
II.	duration	6	bilateral mild disease
III.	duration	7	bilateral disease with early impairment of postural stability
IV.	duration	9	severe disease requiring considerable assistance
V.	duration	14	confinement to bed or wheelchair unless aided

*median duration of illness in years since onset, of patients seen at this stage in 1967, before levodopa therapy.

Before the levodopa era, 28 per cent of patients were disabled (stages IV or V) or dead within 5 years; 61 per cent of those with the disease within 5–10 years; and 83 per cent within 10–15 years. The rate of progression of the disease pathology has probably not been changed by modern dopaminergic drugs. The rate of deterioration of symptoms has however, improved considerably. The proportion of patients reaching stages IV and V is now 9 per cent at 5 years; 22 per cent after 5–10 years; and 55 per cent among those with disease of more than 10 years' duration.[12]

In the pre-levodopa era the average life expectation was about ten years from diagnosis, the longest survivals being in patients with an early age of onset, below the age of 50 (18.4 years). However, only one in four patients survived to 75. Since levodopa the average age at death has increased from 67 to 73 years, and nearly 60 per cent survive to 75 years.

In deciding treatments, these data are pertinent. Patients now seldom die directly of their disease, but succumb to incidental heart attacks, strokes, and neoplasia, or to the sequelae of immobility—urinary infections, decubitus ulcers, and especially the complications of trauma and surgery—not forgetting Osler's 'pneumonia, the friend of the aged'. The wise physician may recognize the need to curtail dopaminergic and other toxic drugs in the preterminal phase when dependency is clearly irreversible.

References

1. Selby, G. (1984). The long term prognosis of Parkinson's disease. *Clinical and Experimental Neurology*, **20**, 1–25.
2. Cody, F. W. J., McDermott, N., Matthews, P. B. C. *et al.* (1986). Observations on the genesis of the stretch reflex in Parkinson's disease. *Brain*, **109**, 229–49.
3. Marsden, C. D. (1990). Neurophysiology. In *Parkinson's disease*, (ed. G. Stern), pp. 57–98. Chapman and Hall, London.
4. Cox, J. G. C., Pearce, I., Steiger, M., and Pearce, J. M. S. (1988). Disordered axial movement in Parkinson's disease. In Parkinson's disease, (ed. F. C. Rose), pp. 71–5. Pitman, London.
5. Marsden, C. D. (1982). The mysterious motor function of the basal ganglia. *Neurology*, **32**, 514–39.
6. Rascol, O., Clanet, M., Montastruc, J. L. *et al.* (1989). Abnormal ocular movements in Parkinson's disease. *Brain*, **112**, 1193–214.
7. Aranda, B., Perrigot, M., Mazieres, L., *et al.* (1983). Les troubles vésico-sphinctériens de la maladie Parkinson. *Revue Neurologique*, **139**(4), 283–8.
8. Brown, R. G., Jahanshahi, M., Quinn, N., and Marsden, C. D. (1990). Sexual function in patients with Parkinson's disease and their partners. *Journal of Neurology, Neurosurgery, and Psychiatry* **53**, 480–7.
9. Doty, R. L., Deems, D. A., and Steller, S. (1988). Olfactory dysfunction in parkinsonism: a general deficit, unrelated to neurologic signs, disease state, or disease duration. *Neurology*, **38**, 1237–44.
10. Inzelberg, R., Treves, T., Reider, I., *et al.* (1987). Computed tomography brain changes in Parkinsonian dementia. *Neuroradiology*, **29**, 535–9.
11. Huber, S. J., Shuttleworth, E. C., Christy, J. A., *et al.* (1989). Magnetic resonance imaging in dementia of Parkinson's disease. *Journal of Neurology, Neurosurgery, and Psychiatry*, **52**, 1221–7.
12. Hoehn, M. M. and Yahr, M. D. (1967). Parkinsonism: onset, progression and mortality. *Neurology*, **17**, 427–42.
13. Hoehn, M. M. (1985). The result of chronic levodopa therapy and its modification by Bromocriptine in Parkinson's disease. *Acta Neurologica Scandinavica*, **71**, 97–106.

5 Classification and differential diagnosis of parkinsonism

Diagnoses are missed not because of lack of knowledge on the part of the examiner, but rather because of lack of examination.

Sir William Osler

Differential diagnosis

It is sensible to separate the disease described by James Parkinson (type 1) from a group of disorders which although they affect the same functions and in broad terms the same areas of the brain, are caused by other pathological or metabolic aberrations of the mesostriatal dopaminergic system. This second group are called *secondary* or *symptomatic parkinsonism*. We recognize several types (Table 5.1), and will consider the main issues which are important in clinical differential diagnosis. It is no longer acceptable to diagnose Parkinson's disease without a thorough clinical dissection of the varied clinical patterns which may be obscuring some other illness with a different prognosis, and, more crucially, a different treatment.

The clinician's first problem is to separate Parkinson's disease from symptomatic neuronal degenerations, and from other cerebral lesions including pseudo-parkinsonism. (Table 5.1).

Table 5.1 Clinical differential diagnosis

Clinical problem	Examples
Other types of parkinsonism:	post-encephalitic (rare); drug-induced; neuronal-system degenerations.
Other causes of tremor:	benign familial tremor; thyrotoxicosis; alcoholism.
Other brain disease causing an akinetic–rigid syndrome:	multiple strokes; MS; tumours; Alzheimer's disease; communicating hydrocephalus (see Fig 5.1); neuronal-system degenerations.

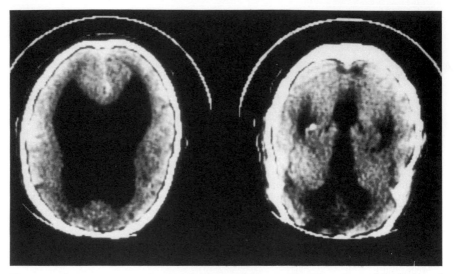

Fig. 5.1 Gross communicating hydrocephalus with dilatation of lateral and third ventricles on CT scan.

Idiopathic paralysis agitans (Parkinson's disease)

Idiopathic ('a cloak for ignorance') means no more than 'the cause is not yet understood'. The hallmarks are degeneration of neuromelanin-containing nerve cells of the midbrain and the presence of Lewy bodies. This is the most common group, comprising probably 90 per cent of all parkinsonian syndromes. Table 5.2 shows a classification of the other major categories of parkinsonism.

Drug-induced parkinsonism

A number of patients (5–7 per cent) suffer from parkinsonism which is due to the long-term use of certain drugs which block the passage of the nerve impulse by blocking the release or transmission of dopamine in the substantia nigra and striatum. These are mainly neuroleptic drugs used for treatment of schizophrenia and other psychoses. Fluorinated phenothiazines (for example, trifluoperazine, fentazine) are more potent than the simpler molecules of promazine and thioridazine; but all of them are culpable. Those most frequently used are shown in Table 5.2, and include those given by injection as a depot.

  Some of these drugs are used (commonly without good indications) to counter nausea, vomiting, or dizziness, and in these circumstances

Table 5.2 Classification of parkinsonism

---

1. Drug-induced parkinsonism
(a) presynaptic blockers, for example, reserpine
(b) post-synaptic receptor blockers, for example, phenothiazines
(c) toxins, for example, CO, Mn, MPTP

2. Post-encephalic parkinsonism

3. Neuronal-system degeneration
(a) multiple-system atrophy
(b) Shy–Drager syndrome
(c) olivopontocerebellar atrophy
(d) progressive supranuclear palsy (Steele–Richardson–Olszewski syndrome)
(e) striatonigral degeneration
(f) cortico–basal degeneration with neuronal achromasia
(g) familial parkinsonism $+/-$ depression
(h) Guam disease (parkinsonism $+/-$ dementia $+/-$ motor-neuron disease
(i) juvenile Parkinson's disease (Ramsay Hunt)

4. Pseudo-parkinsonism
(a) vascular/arteriosclerotic with multi-infarcts
(b) communicating hydrocephalus
(c) brain tumours
(d) traumatic encephalopathy (boxer's brain)

---

parkinsonism should not develop if the course of treatment is restricted to *less than a month* for these symptoms. If the physician is able to withdraw the drugs (Table 5.3) soon after the onset of symptoms the parkinsonism will usually, though not always, slowly disappear, though this may take several months.

Some patients with serious psychiatric illness need to continue the neuroleptic drugs, and some degree of parkinsonism then has to be tolerated to maintain mental stability, and can usually be controlled. Drug-induced parkinsonism may be accompanied by the equally distressing symptoms of

(1) akathisia—compulsive motor restlessness; and

(2) tardive dyskinesia and tardive dystonia, which are often intractable.

These phenomena are not well understood, but are in part dependent on post-synapatic receptor hypersensitivity which is induced by chronic receptor blockade. Excessive sprouting of terminal neuronal vesicles may widen the field of dopaminergic innervation, and the overflow of dopamine metabolites and possibly the so-called 'false neuro-transmitters' into this expanded neural territory may be responsible for the adventitious movements observed. They will not be considered further.

Most patients would probably develop parkinsonian features if treated with a large enough dose of neuroleptic drugs for a sufficient

Table 5.3 Commonly used neuroleptic drugs

---

1. Phenothiazines
chlorpromazine (Largactil)
fluphenazine (Moditen, Motival)
promazine (Sparine)
trifluoperazine (Stelazine)
prochlorperazine (Stemetil)
thioridazine (Melleril), pericyazine (neulactil)
perphenazine (Fentazin, triptafen)

2. Other similar neuroleptic antipsychotic drugs
flupenthixol (Depixol, Fluanxol), zuclopenthixol (Clopixol)
haloperidol (Serenace, Haldol)
droperidol (Droleptan)
*reserpine (Serpasil, Decaserpyl)
*tetrabenazine (Nitoman)
sulpiride (Dolmatil)
pimozide (Orap)

3. Injectable and depot preparations
flupenthixol (Depixol), fluphenazine (Modecate, Moditen), fluspirilene (Redeptin),
Haloperidol (Haldol), pipothiazine (Piportil)

---

*Presynaptic blockers

time. Women seem more susceptible than men, and the incidence is higher in the over-sixties. Symptoms are slow to develop. The physician will often see early signs long before the patient complains: facial masking, loss of arm swing, a slight lack of spontaneous movements and of blinking are all signs of striatal dopamine failure. Later, rigidity, a flexed posture, and resting tremor may emerge, though tremor is less frequent and severe than in Parkinson's disease. Facial expression is reduced, writing becomes smaller, and the small shuffly steps and freezing betray advancing disability as this iatrogenic disease progresses. The signs are generally bilateral, but the distribution can be asymmetrical.

Much rarer are the myoclonic jerks, blepharospasm, and characteristic oculogyric crises, which formerly were diagnostic of post-encephalitic disease. Essentially, the clinical syndrome is indistinguishable from idiopathic Parkinson's disease except for the history of exposure to dopamine-blocking drugs. The commonly prescribed anticholinergic drugs are designed to prevent this drug-induced syndrome, but there is scant evidence that they do so, and they may predispose to tardive dyskinesia and to cognitive impairment. They are better avoided until frank signs emerge. In early cases, with but short exposure to neuroleptic drugs, it sometimes happens that the signs fail to disappear when the drug is withdrawn. In such cases, it is likely that the patient suffers from Parkinson's disease in latent or preclinical form, and that this has been unmasked by the drug-induced state. Less commonly one has encountered patients whose drug-induced state has been reversed by withdrawal, but who years later develop the same picture without further drugs. In these instances, the first illness was clearly a prophecy intimating the later idiopathic disorder.

Patients with drug-induced parkinsonism may respond to anti-cholinergic drugs alone; but others respond inadequately, and levodopa drugs should not then be withheld.

Post-encephalitic parkinsonism

This type of parkinsonism is now extremely rare. It developed in the wake of epidemic encephalitis lethargica (Von Economo's disease)[1] caused by a pandemic of a presumed but unidentified neurotropic virus which raged throughout the world between 1918 and 1926. The polymorphic syndrome[2] comprised a variety of psychic and motor as well as autonomic phenomena. Stupor, hallucinosis, tics, myoclonus, dystonias, oculomotor palsies, and kinetic crises were seen in the evolving illness. Of the two-thirds that recovered, over half progressed to parkinsonism, often many years later. These patients were usually less than 40 years old. They were bradyphrenic and apathetic, and though they often displayed tremor, akinesia, and rigidity, the typical pill-rolling was uncommon, and oculogyric crises, tics, and emotionality were the rule. The disorder often became stationary. It responded better to anticholinergics than to levodopa. I still have two such patients in my care at the time of writing; but what was the second commonest type of parkinsonism has virtually disappeared, though rare instances have occurred sporadically[3] since the great pandemic, which may have caused one million cases world-wide.

Creutzfeldt–Jakob disease (CJD)

This is a transmissible viral encephalopathy with a rapidly fatal course ending in 3 to 6 months. It is characterized by a progressive dementia, myoclonus, stupor, and a variety of multifocal cortical signs. About 10 per cent of cases are familial. Fifteen cases of iatrogenic lateral transmission are recorded,[4] with incubation periods ranging from 16 months to 23 years; there is no sound evidence for casual case-to-case transmission. The agent may be an inherent component of the genome. It contains no nucleic acid, and is classed as an infectious protein or protovirin (prion protein: PrP 27–30), and is similar to the agent found in sheep scrapie and bovine spongiform encephalopathy (BSE), which may replicate in mitochondria. It is a post-transitionally modified isoform of normal precursor proteins, demonstrated by immunostaining of amyloid plaques.

Diagnostic criteria[5] are: a history of rapidly advancing dementia, accompanied by varying combinations of the typical signs of CJD (myoclonus, other movement disorders, cortical blindness, cerebellar ataxia, parkinsonian-type rigidity, akinetic mutism) and histological confirmation of spongiform degeneration. Cases are classed as 'probable' if they have similar clinical features accompanied by an EEG displaying 1–2 Hz triphasic complexes, but with no histology available. Cases are classed as 'possible' if they have the above clinical features but no histology or EEG confirmation.

Hemiparesis, hemianopia, dysarthria, ataxia, and parkinsonian signs are well-recognized consequences of a massive degeneration of cortical neurons, with spongiform vacuolar changes and gliosis.

Gerstmann–Sträusler–Scheinker syndrome

This is closely related to Creutzfeldt–Jakob disease and is usually familial, inherited as an autosomal dominant disorder. The disease has been related to a mutation of the PrP gene at codon 102 similar to those found in familial CJD. The mean age of onset is 40, and it progresses to death in 5 years. Parkinsonism is not a notable feature.

The main signs are: cerebellar ataxia, dementia, nystagmus, scanning speech, pseudobulbar signs, dysaesthesiae in the legs, decreased leg reflexes, and extensor plantar responses. The neuropathology is atrophy of the cortex and cerebellum; multicentric kuru-like plaques are seen in the cerebellum, senile and primitive plaques in the cerebral cortex; and spongiform change, with or without atrophy of long tracts, is found[6].

Parkinsonian rigid–akinetic syndromes and pseudo-parkinsonism

Head injury

These non-specific syndromes result from a variety of other lesions of the brain. Parkinsonism is not normally a feature of **head injury**, though a complex encephalopathy with dementia, dysarthria, ataxia, fits, and pyramidal tract and parkinsonian features characterizes the repeated brain injury of certain boxers ('boxer's brain' or dementia pugilistica). The signs extend beyond the basal ganglia, and are best regarded as 'pseudo-parkinsonism'. Pathologically these avoidable illnesses show old petechial haemosiderin deposits in tiny lacunae in the cortex and brain stem, with plaques and fibrillary tangles and degenerative nerve-cell loss and gliosis involving the cortex and basal nuclei.[7] **Litigation** claims after road and industrial injuries are common, but individually the case for the head injury as the cause of parkinsonism is less than convincing. In some patients the disease has been present in mild or latent form before the injury, which has merely drawn attention to it. Family witnesses are unlikely to testify accurately or objectively to the pre-accident state in these financially-loaded circumstances. Most surveys in the literature[8] have failed to provide convincing data. The pathology and clinical features portrayed have often been exiguous and inadequate for any firm opinon about causality. Exceptional case reports[9] do indicate a causal role on very rare occasions, but the head injury has always been of great severity with prolonged coma; other physical signs indicate that this is one form of pseudo-parkinsonism.

Brain tumours

Brain tumours and subdural haematomas seldom cause parkinsonian syndromes, though occasional parasaggital meningiomata or deep thalamic or corpus callosum tumours can impair basal ganglia function and produce a rigid akinetic syndrome indistinguishable in its early days from Parkinson's disease. Investigations with CT are indicated in younger subjects, those with a rapidly progressing illness, those with non-parkinsonian physical signs, and those who are unresponsive to therapy.

Cerebrovascular disease

As a cause of parkinsonism this condition was grotesquely over-diagnosed, especially in the elderly. Most such cases had a multi-infarct state, with bilateral stiffness, bradykinesia, and *marche à petit pas*; but their signs were due in the main to pyramidal tract damage without lesions in the nigrostriatum. Many are hypertensive, and often they show pseudobulbar palsy in varying degree. Thus their dribbling and dysphonia were mistaken for the clinically different bulbar signs of Parkinson's disease. It is extremely rare to have a demonstrated nigral or putaminal infarct with a parkinsonian syndrome caused thereby, though of course the non-causal coincidence of parkinsonism with vascular disease and infarcts on CT or MRI is quite frequent, as might be expected in two common disorders. Most agree with Toole[10] 'Athero-sclerosis *per se* cannot cause parkinsonism. In the patients whose syndrome resembles parkinsonism, there is associated pyramidal dysfunction, dementia, and/or pseudobulbar signs in addition to the extrapyramidal disorder . . . lacunar state is often found at autopsy.'

The Hachinski score is often applied in an attempt to identify the cause of dementia as vascular, Alzheimer's disease, or both; similar principles are relevant to parkinsonism, but in practice not applicable. Both cerebrovascular disease and Parkinson's disease are common in later life, and their concurrence is often coincidental rather than causal. Binswanger's disease, with its characteristic but non-specific periventricular leukoaraiosis on CT, may cause pseudo-parkinsonism in addition to progressive dementia and multifocal ischaemic symptoms, usually in a hypertensive subject. Atherosclerotic changes and hyalinosis of small arteries and arterioles of the deep white matter are the pathological basis.

Other tremulous states

Other tremulous states need to be excluded. Alcoholism, hyperthyroidism, and liver and renal failure as well as drug dependency and anxiety states can usually be distinguished in the clinic with a minimum of investigation.

Benign essential (familial) tremor causes more diagnostic confusion. It is very common and benign, though of nuisance value, and can start at any age. Most commonly it is first noticed between the ages of 20 and 40. It is a postural tremor, often absent at rest but obvious when the arms are held outstretched. The voice and head are often affected, the legs rarely. Posture is normal and, though some show some signs of 'cogwheeling', true lead-pipe rigidity is absent and, most importantly, spontaneous and voluntary movements are unimpaired. Relief from small amounts of alcohol and a postive family history are typical but not invariable features. Many patients improve with β-blocking drugs.

Neuronal system degeneration

Multiple-system atrophy (Shy–Drager syndrome)

This condition usually presents to the neurologist in a middle-aged patient with varying mixtures of

(1) an akinetic rigid syndrome with tremor absent or inconspicuous;

(2) autonomic failure—impotence and incontinence; and

(3) cerebellar ataxia, and in some cases isolated laryngeal abductor paralysis.[11,12]

The patients fail to obtain much benefit from levodopa drugs and the condition progresses. After two or more years fainting begins, and abnormalities of sweating and impotence may be noted. Minor autonomic abnormalities are not uncommon in classic Parkinson's disease, so that early diagnosis is difficult. Orthostatic hypotension, incontinence, or male impotence may be the only presenting symptoms,[13] and the parkinsonian features show later. Posturally-induced cerebral ischaemic symptoms—flashing lights, hemianopia, amaurosis, vertigo, dysarthria, and paraesthesiae—may be confused with athero-thrombotic TIAs. Investigations of supine and erect blood pressure, thermal sweating, pressor tests, and Valsalva's manoeuvre are required. All the anti-parkinsonian drugs may aggravate these symptoms. Hypotension may be partially controlled by tight anti-embolic stockings, fludrocortisone, and in some patients indomethacin or alpha adrenergic drugs. Antigravity suits have occasionally been used in refractory cases, but they are cumbersome and ill-tolerated. Good symptomatic control is not possible in some patients despite these measures.

Olivopontocerebellar atrophy

This condition should be suscepted in patients presenting parkinsonian signs at an early age (for example, < 50 years) who have additional signs of ataxia, brisk reflexes, and extensor plantar responses. Chorea or athetosis may be evident, though unsteadiness due to ataxia is the most common initial finding. Eye movements of limited extent on voluntary gaze or pursuit with preserved doll's-eye movements suggests a supra-nuclear disorder. Cerebellar disease may be suspected if on distant fixation of an object for a minimum of 10 seconds, the eyes show abrupt irregular jerks (square-wave jerks), a sign of instability of fixation. Defective visual suppression of the normal vestibulo–ocular reflex can be easily demonstrated. The eyes are fixed on the end of a tendon hammer when the rubber end is applied and held to the forehead. The patient stares at the end and the examiner slowly rotates the head to either side. In the abnormal responses the eyes are seen to lag behind repeatedly, and then to jerk into the corrected position.

The family history is positive in some but by no means all cases of this heterogeneous symptom complex. Response to dopamine drugs is usually poor.

Progressive supranuclear palsy (Steele, Richardson, Olszewski)

This rare disorder is seldom recognized at presentation. Slowness of movement, rigidity, and akinesia are the initial symptoms in most patients. The first lady I recognized as having this disorder was a nurse who kept tripping and falling. Careful enquiry as to why she tripped provoked the interesting comment that she could not focus on the ground for about three yards in front of her. Examination showed impaired conjugate vertical gaze, both up and down, so that she failed to see obstacles, kerbs, and carpet edges immediately in front of her; the falling was thus explained. The characteristic signs are defects of conjugate supranuclear gaze, often first in the downward plane; upward gaze and later lateral gaze are also affected. Oculo-kinetic responses and doll's-eye responses are often preserved, and confirm the supranuclear pattern. Nystagmus is not apparent, and pupils are normal at presentation. Many show a distinctive 'stare' due to mild lid retraction. These patients do not show the flexed posture of the parkinsonian, and indeed are often notably erect. Later the neck may even appear retracted in extension dystonia. Dysarthria is common, and may progress to virtual anarthria. Pseudobulbar signs emerge with pathological laughter and crying, dribbling, and masking of the face due to spasticity. Reflexes are normal or brisk, and the plantars may be extensor.

The patients do not respond well to dopamine drugs,[14] though I can confirm reports that a slight amelioration may be obtained for a brief time.

CT or MRI scans may be normal in the early stages of the illness, but later high-resolution scans will show atrophy of the pontine and midbrain tegmentum and a widened aqueduct of Sylvius. Fronto-temporal atrophy may be present. The disease is progressive, with an average period of 5 to 8 years from diagnosis to death.

Striato-nigral degeneration

There is no reliable diagnostic clinical picture for this syndrome. It is suspected if a patient presents without the characteristic rest tremor but has an akinetic rigid syndrome which proves refractory to therapy with dopaminergic drugs. This may amount to about one third of those 10 per cent of patients who appear to display primary failure to respond to levodopa.[15]

Cortico-basal degeneration

This is also a pathologically-defined syndrome which is clinically indistinct. Examples with neuronal achromasia have recently been described—perhaps another hint of the special significance of neuronal pigments in relationship to degenerative diseases.[16] In addition to bradykinesia, rigidity, and possibly tremor, the early presence of cognitive defects and hyper-reflexia and Babinski signs should arouse suspicion.

Familial parkinsonism

This condition is always striking, and self-evident provided that the allegedly affected relatives can be meticulously examined. When this is not possible every means should be sought to obtain and to validate the clinical records of other physicians. Confusion with olivopontocerebellar atrophy and benign familial (syn.: 'essential') tremor is common; the distinction should be clearly made before the diagnosis of familial parkinsonism is accepted. There are interesting families with proven examples of both essential tremor and Parkinson's disease in different members. To add to the confusion, one has encountered individuals with essential tremor since their early twenties or thirties who have later shown unequivocal Parkinson's disease. Since the prevalence of essential tremor is 2–4 per cent in the over-forties in the community, this is not entirely surprising.

Guam disease

This well-reported triad of sinister neurological ailments—Parkinsonism, motor neuron disease, and presenile dementia—remains endemic to the Chamorro tribe in Guam. There is no known causal link between this illness and the occasional unfortunate individual seen in Britain and the USA who develops both MND and Parkinson's disease. Dementia may additionally complicate a significant minority of Parkinson's disease victims.

Juvenile parkinsonism

Ramsay Hunt in 1917 described four patients with juvenile paralysis agitans, and the autopsy of one whose illness started at the age of 15 and who died aged 40.[17] Two earlier cases were reported by Siehr in 1899.[18] The clinical features described by Hunt were similar to adult cases: the pathology consisted of 'chronic atrophy and decreased numbers of neurons and increased glial cells in the globus pallidus, putamen and caudate nucleus'. The substantia nigra was 'normal'. One of the four patients developed pyramidal signs, and died aged 65. Davison[19] reported the pathological findings 'the same as in parkinsonism except . . . for demyelination of the pyramidal tracts within the medulla oblongata and spinal cord'. The substantia nigra was shrunk and depigmented. On microscopic examination; there was extensive cellular loss. Van Bogaert[19] described a 7-year-old with tremor, rigidity, and pseudobulbar signs prior to death at the age of 30; the major pathology was atrophy of the globus pallidus. Martin *et al.*[20] described two brothers presenting classical parkinsonian signs at the ages of 10 and 16; they responded well to levodopa. Their paternal grandfather's brother had drug-induced parkinsonism. Subsequent cases[21] have shown classical parkinsonian signs, in some a familial—possibly autosomal dominant—basis, a prolonged course, and a response to levodopa drugs. I have currently in my care a 52-year-old man with classic disease onset at 15, and a 48-year-old man with an onset at the age of 27. Neither have a family history, both respond well to levodopa and one of them responds to dopamine agonist drugs. Whether this juvenile syndrome is the young end of the spectrum of adult disease, or is an aetiologically different disease, manifesting similar clinical stigmata, remains an enigma.

Conclusion

The differential diagnosis of the syndrome embraces a wide variety of other cerebral lesions. Spot diagnosis in the clinic is still a valid basis for the diagnosis of a parkinsonian syndrome, but it is no longer a complete or adequate description of the diagnosis, nor of the prognosis and likely outcome of treatment. Since over 15 per cent of patients diagnosed as having Parkinson's disease in life prove to have other diagnoses, the clinician should be vigilant and should sedulously search for unseen or unsuspected features.

Diagnosis of Parkinson's disease: suggested new criteria

The neuropathological hallmarks of idiopathic Parkinson's disease are Lewy bodies in the pigmented neuromelanin cells of the substantia nigra (SN) and other brain-stem nuclei, and fallout of neurons in the SN, with degeneration of the nigrostriatal pathway.

The Cambridge-based 'brain-bank' has shown that the traditional clinical criteria for the diagnosis of Parkinson's disease are unreliable, with errors in between 15 and 20 per cent of patients.

Errors commonly arise from the mixed extrapyramidal disorders presenting (see Tables 5.1 and 5.2), and more specifically those conditions listed in Table 5.4.

Many patients have distinctive associated features additional to parkinsonism which should arouse suspiscion. Examples include the

Table 5.4 Differential diagnosis

---

1. Benign (sometimes familial) essential tremor
2. Multi-infarct states
3. Alzheimer's disease complicated by extrapyramidal signs (in up to 60 per cent of cases)
4. Multi-system atrophy (MSA), including the Shy–Drager syndrome
5. Olivopontocerebellar atrophy (OPCA)
6. Progressive supranuclear palsy (Steele–Richardson–Olszewski syndrome)
7. Diffuse (cortical and brain-stem) Lewy-body disease
8. Striatonigral degeneration
9. Cortico–striatal (cortico–basal) degeneration
10. Others: neuroleptics, tumours, vascular disease, infective encephalitides, and so on

---

paresis of vertical gaze in progressive supranuclear palsy, the impotence and orthostatic hypotension in multi-system atrophy, the history of multiple strokes, or TIAs in multi-infarct states. But in the early stages these features may be inconspicuous; errors in diagnosis may become apparent only with the passage of time and the late emergence of associated physical signs. The prognosis and response to treatment in these patients with parkinsonism differ significantly from those of Parkinson's disease; hence the importance of their recognition.

Diagnostic accuracy is improved by taking the following steps (Table 5.7):

1. Establish the presence of parkinsonism, using traditional criteria (Table 5.5).

2. Exclude causes of symptomatic and pseudo-parkinsonism (Tables 5.1, 5.2, and 5.4).

3. Confirm the presence of the more specific features of Parkinson's disease (Table 5.6) and supplement this if necessary by the levodopa and/or apomorphine tests (see p. 50).

Additional and possibly predictive criteria may be gained from the levodopa and apomorphine tests.

A. Levodopa test

1. All therapy stopped for 24 hours.

2. Clinical rating scale at -30 mins and 0 hour.

3. Fasting at 8–9 a.m. Oral levodopa 400 mg + benserazide 50 mg as madopar (2×250 mg tablets), or levodopa 500 mg + carbidopa 50 mg as sinemet (2×275 mg tablets), *statim*.

4. Repeat clinical rating scale at peak of improvement, usually between 45 and 150 mins.

5. A positive response is a 25 per cent improvement.

Table 5.5 Traditional criteria of parkinsonism (syn.: parkinsonian syndrome)

1. Bradykinesia, plus one of the following
2. Resting tremor, 4–6 Hz
3. Rigidity, usually lead-pipe or cogwheel, in limbs, neck, or trunk
4. Postural instability, not of visual, vestibular, cerebellar, or proprioceptive origin.

Table 5.6 Parkinson's disease: suggested revised criteria

Three or more of the following features:
1. At onset: slow, 4–6 Hz, resting tremor in one or more limbs **plus one or more signs of:**
2. Predominantly unilateral distribution at onset.
3. Rigidity—lead-pipe or cogwheel (in axial muscles or limbs), plus hypokinesia or bradykinesia of face, trunk, or limb movement, including gait; postural abnormalities.
4. A substantial and unequivocal clinical response (33–100 per cent reduction of clinical rating scales to levodopa treatment within 2 months.[22,23]

B. Apomorphine test

1. All therapy stopped for 24 hours; give oral domperidone 20 mg × 8 hourly.

2. Clinical rating scale at − 30 minutes and 0 hour.

3. At 0 hour give subcutaneous apomorphine 2 mg *stat.*

4. Repeat clinical rating scale at 30, 60, and 120 mins.

5. A positive response is a 25 per cent improvement.

6. If negative, repeat using 3 mg, 5 mg, and 10 mg at 4-hourly intervals until a positive response is observed.

We use the Webster clinical rating test (10 items, maximum score 30); but other standardized motor scales can be used. Excellent agreement has been found between the initial challenges with levodopa and apomorphine. Apomorphine also predicts the response to long-term levodopa therapy in 90 per cent (58/65) of patients[22] with Parkinson's disease.

The use of the clinical criteria supplemented by a positive levodopa or apomorphine test has refined the diagnosis of idiopathic Parkinson's disease in our clinic. Negative and equivocal tests suggest the other parkinsonian syndromes (Table 5.1), and thereby assist prognosis and anticipation of the results of treatment. Errors will result if too much reliance is placed on the levodopa or apomorphine tests if used without detailed clinical analysis (as above) since positive results may sometimes be seen in PSP, MSA, and mixed dementia and parkinsonism (many corresponding to diffuse Lewy-bodies disease) and in other mixed basal-ganglia syndromes. Some of these are at least in part responsive to levodopa therapy. I have seen patients with MSA diagnosed up to 6 years after typical Parkinson's disease conforming to the above criteria, who still showed resting tremor and dose-related dyskinesia with a good response to each dose of sinemet. Thus a positive test is a reliable indication of a dopamine-responsive syndrome, and a negative test argues strongly against established idiopathic Parkinson's disease.

A proposed schema is shown in Table 5.7 to clarify the steps necessary in reaching a diagnosis of idiopathic Parkinson's disease. No doubt, with time and with the advent of further refinements in testing, this too will need to be modified.

Table 5.7 Schema for diagnosis of idiopathic Parkinson's disease

1. Diagnose parkinsonism by criteria in Table 5.3.
2. Exclude causes of symptomatic parkinsonism (parkinsonian syndromes (Table 5.4)).
3. Idiopathic Parkinson's disease is probable if clinical criteria conform to Table 5.5. If these criteria are **not** met, the patient is likely to have symptomatic parkinsonism.
4. If the levodopa or apomorphine is positive the probability is increased. A positive test implics dopaminergic responsiveness and predicts a therapeutic response with contined oral therapy.

References

1. Von Economo, C. (1931). *Encephalitis lethargica: its sequelae and treatment.* Oxford University Press, Oxford.
2. Sacks, O. (1973). *Awakenings.* Duckworth, London.
3. Howard, R. S. and Lees, A. J. (1987). Encephalitis lethargica: a report of four recent cases. *Brain,* **110**, 19–33.
4. Cousens, S. N., Harries-Jones, R., Knight, R., *et al.* (1990). Geographical distribution of cases of Creutzfeldt–Jakob disease in England and Wales 1970–84. *Journal of Neurology, Neurosurgery, and Psychiatry,* **53**, 459–65.
5. Will, R. G. and Matthews, W. B. (1984). A retrospective study of Jakob–Creutzfeldt disease in England and Wales, 1970–1979. 1. Clinical features. *Journal of Neurology, Neurosurgery, and Psychiatry,* **47**, 134–40.
6. Hart, J. and Gordon, B. (1990). Early onset of dementia and extra-pyramidal disease: clinicopathological variant of Gerstmann–Strausler–Scheinker or Alzheimer's disease? *Journal of Neurology, Neurosurgery, and Psychiatry,* **53**, 932–4.
7. Mawdsley, C. and Ferguson, F. R. (1963). Neurological disease in boxers. *Lancet,* **2**, 795–801.

8. Koller, W. C., Wong, G. F., and Lang, A. (1989). Post-traumatic movement disorders: a review. *Movement Disorders*, **4**(1), 20–36.

9. Nayermouri, T. (1985). Post-traumatic parkinsonism. *Surgical Neurology*, **24**, 264–6.

10. Toole, J. F. (1990). *Cerebrovascular disease*, (4th edn.) pp. 266–7. Raven Press, New York.

11. Williams, A., Hanson, D., and Calne, D. B. (1979). Vocal cord paralysis in the Shy–Drager syndrome. *Journal of Neurology, Neurosurgery, and Psychiatry*, **42**, 151–3.

12. Kew, J., Gross, M., and Chapman, P. (1990). Shy–Drager syndrome presenting as isolated paralysis of vocal cord abductors. *British Medical Journal*, **300**, 1441.

13. Bannister, R. (1983) *Autonomic failure*, pp. 67–73. Oxford University Press, Oxford.

14. Goetz, C. G., Tanner, C. M., and Klawans, H. L. (1984). The pharmacology of olivopontocerebellar atrophy. *Advances in Neurology*, **41**, 143–8.

15. Rajput, H., Kazi, K. G., and Rozdilski, B. (1972). Striatonigral degeneration: response to levodopa therapy. *Journal of Neurology, Neurosurgery, and Psychiatry*, **16**, 331–41.

16. Gibb, W. R. G., Luthert, P., and Marsden, C. D. (1989). Cortico-basal degeneration. *Brain*, **112**, 1171–92.

17. Hunt, J. R. (1917). Progressive atrophy of the globus pallidus (primary atrophy of the pallidal system); a system disease of paralysis agitans type. *Brain*, **40**: 58–148.

18. Siehr, P. (cited by Sachdev *et al.* (1899). *Zwei falle von paralysis agitans in jugendlichem*. Thesis, Kaliningrad, Russia (Königsberg).

19. Davison, C. (1954). Pallido-pyramidal disease. *Journal of Experimental Neurology*, **13**, 50–9.

20. Martin, W. E., Fesch, J. A., and Baker, A. B. (1971). Juvenile parkinsonism. *Archives of Neurology*, **25**, 494–500.

21. Sachdev, K. K., Singh, N., and Krishnamoorthy, M. S. (1977). Juvenile parkinsonism treated with levodopa. *Archives of Neurology*, **34**, 244–5.

22. Hughes, A. J., Lees, A. J., and Stern, G. M. (1990). Apomorphine test to predict dopaminergic responsiveness in parkinsonian syndromes. *Lancet*, **2**, 32–4.

23. Gibbs, W. R. G. and Lees, A. J. (1988). The relevance of Lewy body disease to the pathogenesis of idiopathic Parkinson's disease. (Table 1. UK Parkinson's Disease Society brain bank clinical diagnostic criteria). *Journal of Neurology, Neurosurgery, and Psychiatry*, **51**, 745–52.

6 Neurotransmitters and diagnostic markers

Neurotransmitters

In recent years the identification and assays of brain neurotransmitters have provided fascinating insights into the existence of chemical circuitry and neuronal systems, illustrations of which are in many ways comparable to the efforts of the traditional anatomical 'diagram makers' whose sedulous application in a different context was so disdained by Head. Figure 6.1 shows a simplified version of the synthesis of dopamine from tyrosine, the transmission across the synaptic cleft, and the critical dopamine receptor sites on the post-synaptic membrane.

Neurotransmitters can be measured and serve as an index of neuronal function. Biochemical measurement in autopsy tissue homogenates is now supplemented by immunocytochemical tests employing specific antibodies directed at single transmitters and their synthesizing enzymes. The common neurochemicals studied include dopaminergic,

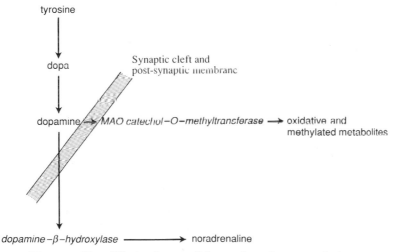

Fig. 6.1 Simplified schema of dopaminergic transmission.

cholinergic, noradrenergic, serotoninergic, and neuropeptidergic systems. Knowledge increases so rapidly that any attempt at a synthesis of current information is quickly outdated.

Dopamine

It is well established that when the first signs of the disease are manifest, dopamine levels are reduced by 80 per cent in the substantia nigra and striatum. The primary deficit lies in the presynaptic dopaminergic neuron where dopamine is stored and then released into the synaptic cleft. Re-uptake of dopamine and other neurotransmitters occurs in the synaptic cleft, enhancing the available dopaminergic stores (Fig. 6.2).This is associated with pathological signs of destruction of a similar proportion of the system of dopaminergic neurons. It is established that there is degeneration of:

(1) the mesostriatal dopaminergic pathway (see Fig. 3.5). Changes are maximum in the putamen.

(2) an ascending dopaminergic pathway from the midbrain ventral tegmentum to the cortex and limbic systems—the meso-cortico-limbic system. This is much less affected than the mesostriatal system.

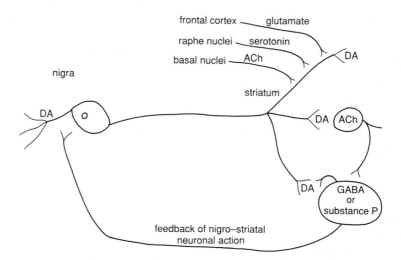

Fig. 6.2 Routes of presynaptic dopaminergic nigro–striatal pathway.

(3) selective dopaminergic hypothalamic nuclei, other neurotransmitters in this area being spared.

(4) dopaminergic neuronal systems in the globus pallidus, locus coeruleus, and amygdala.

Consequences of dopaminergic depletion

Clinical

Clinical responses to levodopa and dopamine agonists, MPTP studies, and studies of primate neurotoxic lesions of the nigra prove that dopamine deficiency is the main factor responsible for the various akinetic features of the ailment. Dopamine deficiency may play a part in the genesis of rigidity and tremor, but precise correlations are lacking. Mesocorticolimbic dopamine depletion may contribute to the mental symptoms of Parkinson's disease, but current evidence leaves this an unresolved problem, especially since levodopa replacement confers no dramatic benefit on this aspect. A general alerting effect and improvement in the bradyphrenia have been claimed.[1,2] The nausea and vomiting of early levodopa therapy has been attributed to stimulation of receptors in the area postrema. These toxic symptoms are largely offset by peripheral dopa decarboxylase inhibitors present in Madopar and Sinemet.

Dyskinesia complicating dopamine therapy is more prominent with levodopa than with direct D2 agonist drugs. It tends to occur after 1 or 2 years of treatment, and is conspicuous at peak dosage when patients are 'on', with lessened parkinsonian signs and disabilities. The end-of-dose dyskinesia is related to falling dopamine levels, when the receptors may be hypersensitive and 'overactive' in an attempt to compensate for waning neurotransmitter levels; this remains speculative. The pattern of oscillations in clinical signs and especially the apparently random nature of their 'on-off' swings late in the disease are not understood (see Chapter 11). Decreased absorption of the drug from the GI tract, inhibition of dopamine by other dietary amino acids (see Chapter 11), and a failure of the central 'buffer mechanism' to both store and release dopamine are all factors.

Experimental

There is some evidence of increased production of dopaminergic metabolites (HVA and DOPAC) relative to the decrease of dopamine in the striatum: the HVA/dopamine ratio. This is interpreted as a sign of increased activity in the remaining dopaminergic cells.

Investigations show variation in neuronal dopaminergic metabolism.[3] The excessive drive in the mesostriatum is not accompanied by corresponding increases in the HVA/dopamine ratio in cortical and limbic projection. This hyperactivity is evident both in neuronal dopamine and in dopaminergic nerve terminals linking the striatum to other basal ganglia and thalamic and limbic areas.

Denervation hypersensitivity

There is increasing information that the density of dopamine receptors is increased in Parkinson's disease. This trend is probably less marked in patients treated with levodopa, which implies that dopamine depletion leads to sprouting of nerve terminals and receptors, and that replacing the deficiency with levodopa inhibits this process. There are two main striatal receptors D1 (adenylate cyclase dependent) and D2, and curiously the latter is not increased in the caudate though it is in the putamen. Data on D1 receptors are contradictory. There may be subsets of striatal neurons which are differentially affected; but further research is needed to clarify these problems.

The consequences of dopamine denervation[4] are compensatory receptor hyperactivity, but in the early phases, before the critical 80 per cent depletion is reached, there is also increased turnover of dopamine in presynaptic neurons which successfully delays the emergence of clinical phenomena. In a later phase there is still no sign of receptor hypersensitivity but the HVA/dopamine ratios increase as a result of presynaptic failure. Clinical signs are present but mild. Patients respond well and predictably to dopamine medication, usually without dyskinesia.

In the advanced state, decompensation occurs: over 80 per cent of dopamine neurons are functionally ineffective, and post-synaptic receptor activity increases. This phase corresponds to the 'on–off' swings, dyskinesias and dystonias, diurnal fluctuations, and unpredictable oscillations which are not clearly related to the timing of oral medication. However, it has been shown that both intravenous levodopa infusions and injections of apomorphine, a direct dopamine receptor agonist, are still effective in averting the off-phase, so that *the receptors are still in large measure responsive*. It is thought that dopamine neurons are now failing adequately to convert levodopa to dopamine. The hypersensitivity of D2 receptors probably explains drug-induced dyskinesia (see Chapters 11 and 12).

Pharmacological strategies at the dopamine synapse

At the dopaminergic synapse, dopamine activity may be increased by several mechanisms in theory.

1. The precursor levodopa may be increased by oral, transduodenal, or intravenous administration.

2. In theory a co-factor could enhance the rate-determining enzyme activity governing the synthesis of dopa from tyrosine.

3. Dopamine release across the synaptic cleft could be enhanced.

4. At the postsynaptic receptor, stimulation results from dopamine agonists (for example, bromocriptine, lisuride, pergolide).

5. Retention of dopamine metabolites may be increased (for example, selegiline).

6. In the synaptic cleft, blockade of the autoreceptor which controls tyrosine hydroxylase.

7. Blockade of dopamine re-uptake into the presynaptic neuron may enhance dopaminergic transmission (Fig. 6.2).

Other neurotransmitter systems

Pathologically, the degenerative lesion and presence of Lewy bodies in the nucleus basalis of Meynert, reticular formation, locus coeruleus, and dorsal vagal nucleus suggest that other ascending neurotransmitter systems will be implicated.

Cholinergic

Choline acetyl transferase (CAT) is the marker for **cholinergic** neuronal function. No consistent reduction in the caudate or nigra has been shown and the muscarinic receptors are apparently normal. The efficacy of anticholinergic drugs is thought to be the result of an excessive cholinergic function, either relative to the dopamine depletion or resulting from the reduction in the normal action of dopamine in inhibiting cholinergic action.

The degeneration of Meynert's nucleus explains the reduction of CAT activity in the neocortex.[5] This is associated with altered cognitive function, particularly memory. In some patients there is coexistent

Alzheimer's disease pathology, with neuronal fall-out, plaques, and neurofibrillary tangles; in others with similar cholinergic denervation of the cortex, no such pathology can be invoked. Early hopes for symptomatic reversal of the dementia in some parkinsonian subjects have so far been unfulfilled. There is some evidence that anticholinergic drugs aggravate the forgetfulness and confusion later in the illness, and it is prudent to withdraw them as the disease advances and in the elderly.

Serotoninergic

Serotoninergic transmitters ascend to the forebrain from the raphe nuclei of the reticular formation. Serotonin (5-HT) and its metabolic breakdown product (5-HIAA) are reduced significantly in the basal ganglia, hypothalamus, hippocampus, and frontal cortex in Parkinson's disease. No gross receptor changes have however been found, and the clinical significance remains uncertain. Drugs increasing 5-HT do not affect tremor. A role for 5-HT deficiency in depression has been claimed, and serotoninergic imipramine binding receptors are decreased.

Noradrenergic

The locus coeruleus is a prime source of the noradrenergic (NA) ascending system. The synthetic NA enzyme is dopamine-β-hydroxylase (DBH), which acts as a marker for noradrenergic cells. Concentrations of NA, DBH, and the metabolites of NA are markedly reduced in the cortex, where there is an increased density of post-synaptic β receptor sites as a result of cortical denervation. Loss of the ascending pathway appears to be partial and patchy, other adrenergic receptors being spared.

   The clinical significance is uncertain. Speculation has it that NA depletion might affect other neurotransmitters, including dopamine. A contributory role in akinesia and freezing has also been postulated. Tricyclic drugs improve both depression and to some extent other motor functions, so that problems in these areas have been seen as at least partially the result of noradrenergic deficiency.

Neuropeptides

Neuronal degeneration in basal ganglia has been accompanied by reduced levels of neuropeptides. There are five neuropeptides of interest: met-enkephalin, leu-enkephalin, somatostatin, substance P, and cholecystokinin. There is unfortunately insufficient basis to allow correlation of these findings with clinical symptomatology, though the fairly selective depletion of somatostatin in the cortex may relate to the dementia found in about 10 to 20 per cent of patients.[6] The inhibitory GABA system may also be depleted, as shown by reduced glutamic acid decarboxylase (GAD) levels; but measurements are influenced by agonal changes, and are therefore not reliable.

Conclusion

The principal abnormality remains that of severe and progressive striatal dopamine depletion. It is known that normal nigrostriatal function utilizes dopamine to effect the fine tuning of motor control (Chapter 4). Dopamine deficiency leads to a major part if not the whole mechanism of breakdown of the motor system in Parkinson's disease.

Diagnostic markers

As with certain other diseases, there are no specific or diagnostic tests which confirm or refute the diagnosis. Routine biochemical and haematological tests and electroencephalograms (EEG) are essentially normal.

A search for diagnostic markers in theory aims at:

(1) confirming the diagnosis;

(2) finding perhaps a measure of disease activity which could be used to monitor (a) progression and (b) the effects of treatment; and

(3) detecting preclinical disease which might in turn be responsive to treatment.

In practice what follows is a catalogue of substantially negative or non-specific abnormalities; no good diagnostic marker yet exists.

Computed tomography (CT) commonly shows cortical atrophy, ventricular dilatation, and coincident vascular infarction; but these signs are non-specific, and the role of aging alone is responsible for much of the 'radiological atrophy' often demonstrated.[7] Similarly, magnetic resonance imaging (MRI) shows no consistent change from control subjects in respect of surface area of the brain, ventricular measurements, number of supratentorial and infratentorial lesions, and signal brightness and width of the substantia nugra.[8] Other workers have reported reduction of width and signal intensity from the nigra.

Positron emission tomographic (PET) scans permit measurements of regional distribution of administered radionuclides and produce an autoradiograph. The application of [^{18}F] 6-fluorodopa produces an index of dopaminergic metabolism; the administration of [^{76}Br]-bromospiperone shows D2 receptor density, and distribution and [^{11}C]-raclopide has been investigated to show receptor binding in the striatum and after neural grafts. So far, no consistent abnormalities of diagnostic value have been obtained. Findings of research interest are likely in the near future, but it is a highly complex, expensive, and specialized technique which is unlikely to be suited to routine use in a common disorder.

Homovanillic acid is one of the major breakdown products of dopamine. It is found in reduced amounts in the CSF of patients, but there is a big overlap between normal individuals (20–40 mg/ml) and patients (0–20 mg/ml) which, apart from the inconvenience of lumbar puncture, makes this assay unsuitable for clinical purposes. Similarly, reduced hydroxylase cofactors show considerable overlap with levels in control subjects.

Mitochondrial complex 1 is reduced in nigral cells and also in platelets. Whether this is the result or cause of free oxygen and hydroxyl radicals and of iron deposition in the nigra is not known (see Chapter 3). Its measurement is inapplicable as a marker of the disease. The availability of copper and iron in preclinical stages is of interest, but neither are good markers, since normal values are often found in patients.

A search for Free Radical Markers has been made using diene conjugates, TBA reactivity, and reduced ascorbic acid as markers of lipid peroxides. They have been disappointingly non-specific and are poor markers of the disease.

Indices of normal metabolic processes in basal ganglia nuclei have been set up and tested: for example, of hydroxylation, which is a vital step in the synthesis of dopamine by tyrosine hydroxylase. If the population contains good and bad metabolizers (akin to INH) then a group of the latter would be more susceptible in theory to any toxin in the environment. According to 'catastrophe theory', a small change in exposure can then produce a major change causing significant pathology. The metabolic rate of Debrisoquine has been used as an index of hydroxylation, but abnormal results were found not only in parkinsonian but in normal subjects and those with motor neuron disease and Alzheimer's disease.

Sulphur oxidation of l-cysteine has been assessed, and is abnormal in Alzheimer's disease, motor neuron disease, and certain other neurological disorders. The ratio of cysteine to sulphate is increased in Parkinson's disease, but also in Alzheimer's disease and motor neuron disease.

Researchers have sought signs of other impaired metabolic processes which might disclose a basis for impaired detoxification of hitherto unknown poisons in the environment and diet. Thiol methyl transferase detoxifies hydrogen sulphide, which has cyanide-like neurotoxic properties. Levels of this enzyme in Parkinson's disease fall at the lower end of the normal range; but this finding is non-specific, since there are also abnormal results in other neurodegenerative processes. Similarly, a paracetamol test to investigate liver conjugative processes was found to show reduced activity in Parkinson's disease, but also in motor-neuron disease and Alzheimer's disease.

Monoamine oxidase B is the enzyme which changes environmental MPTP to MPDP, which in turn becomes MPP^+, the highly toxic metabolite that causes experimental Parkinson's disease. Measurement of MAOB activity in Parkinson's disease is logical: it has been found to be normal or slightly elevated in peripheral blood, but reduced in platelets. This is of some interest, since reduced levels might indicate consumption of the enzyme in the nigrostriatal pathways.

Conclusion

Further studies are necessary but no useful marker so far has been discovered. The elucidation of these diverse disorders has, however, increased speculation that a linked, genetically-determined metabolic defect may lead to an increased susceptibility to environmental poisons yet to be discovered.

References

1. Lees, A. J. and Smith, E. (1983). Cognitive defects in the early stages of Parkinson's disease. *Brain*, **106**, 257–70.
2. Brown, R. G., Marsden, C. D., Quinn, N., *et al.* (1984). Alterations in cognitive performance can affect arousal state during fluctuations in motor function in Parkinson's disease. *Journal of Neurology, Neurosurgery, and Psychiatry*, **47**, 454–65.
3. Rinne, U. K., Rinne, J. O., Rinne, J. K., *et al.*, (1984). Brain neurotransmitters and neuropeptides in Parkinson's disease. *Acta Physiological Pharmacologica Latinoameticana*, **34**, 287–99.
4. Bokobza, B., Ruberg, M., Scatton, B., *et al.*, (1984). 3H-spiperone binding, dopamine and HVA concentrations in Parkinson's disease and supranuclear palsy. *European Journal of Pharmacology*, **99**, 167–75.
5. Perry, R. H., Tomlinson, B. E., Candy, J. M. *et al.*, (1986). Cortical cholinergic deficit in mentally impaired parkinsonian patients. *Lancet*, **2**, 789–90.

6. Agid, Y., Ruberg, M., Raisman, R., *et al.* (1990). The biochemistry of Parkinson's disease. In *Parkinson's disease*, (ed. G. Stern), pp. 99–126. Chapman and Hall, London.

7. Pearce, J. M. S., Flowers, K., Pearce, I., and Pratt, A. E. (1981). Clinical, psychometric and CAT scan correlations in Parkinson's disease. In *Research progress in Parkinson's disease*, (ed. F. C. Rose and R. Capildeo), pp. 43–52. Pitman, London.

8. Huber, S. J., Shuttleworth, E. C., Christy, J. A. *et al.* (1989). Magnetic resonance imaging in dementia of Parkinson's disease. *Journal of Neurology, Neurosurgery, and Psychiatry*, **52**, 1221–7.

7 Neuropsychological aspects of Parkinson's disease

Nervous and emotional factors play their part in all human disease. The effects of worry and sleeplessness in worsening pain are as well known as the harmful effects of personal worries on the symptoms of, for example, asthma or a stomach ulcer. Conversely, a physical illness such as a fracture, a disk prolapse, or Parkinson's disease not surprisingly engenders anxiety, apprehension, and depression in some patients. Tremor and ponderous slow movements are a source of social embarassment. An abnormal gait, trips and falls, difficulty with speech and voice—each adds to the inconvenience and ultimately can cause grave disability. The fear of dependence on others is ever-present.

These are all subjective and variable effects not specifically related to Parkinson's disease, but invariably related to any chronic and progressive physical illness. The individual's reaction depends on his or her personal resilience and motivation, and of course on a widely variable past lifetime of experiences and on the ever-important genetic substrate. We therefore separate a variety of emotional, affective, and behavioural problems which are more specific to the nature of the illness and which depend in large measure on the defects in the brain: pathological, physiological, and neurochemical. These constitute an integral part of Parkinson's disease. They are extremely important in determining the response to treatment.

Premorbid stage

It is often said that there is a personality type which is recognizable and which precedes the onset of symptoms. There is of course a prolonged period of unknown duration, possibly of ten years or more, in which there is an insidious fallout of nigral cells and a corresponding diminution of endogenous dopamine. That such organic factors could underlie subtle cognitive and behavioural changes should occasion no surprise. Parkinson commented on the 'unhappy sufferer', and cites a case of a Dr Marty who commented 'a more melancholy object I never beheld.' But Parkinson had little personal contact with the objects of his meticulous observation, and concluded 'the senses and intellect are uninjured'. Charcot recognized emotional and genetic factors in the causation of the illness; and subsequent authors have invoked conflict, unresolved stress, and a variety of tension states as aetiological factors. Psychiatrists and analysts have described tense, emotional, repressed introverts with inflexible and unbending attitudes—excessively self-disciplined, the acme of serious and staunch dedication. Similar profiles have been mooted in migraine, asthma, and ulcerative colitis. More formal personality inventories carried out by patients and their spouses on behaviour before the illness has been diagnosed, have however lent some support to this picture.[1]

The tendency for parkinsonian patients to be non-smokers has also been linked to personality types—a situation similar to that in ulcerative colitis. Whether smoking protects against the accumulation of toxic-free radicals or is a marker for a personality type which is more vulnerable to other causal agents remains unknown, but is a fascinating field for speculation.

Depression

A depressive illness occurs at some time in about one-third of all Parkinson's disease patients. By illness is implied symptoms out of proportion to the underlying psychological cause, or symptoms of such severity that the patient cannot cope with them. Depression can occur out of the blue when there is no apparent stress, source of anxiety, or physical disability to explain it; this is *endogenous* depression. It is of interest that the incidence of depression is higher than in the non-parkinsonian population even before the physical signs of Parkinson's disease are apparent. Sufferers feel miserable, unhappy, and low in spirits; they are apathetic: devoid of vitality, interests, and enthusiasms. They push themselves to make the effort to do everyday tasks: getting dressed, shaving, going out, mixing socially, or even having a chat with family or friends. Life seems pointless, hopeless, and futile. Sleep is disturbed. Patients go to bed early to get away from it all, sleep fitfully till 4 or 5 in the morning, and then can sleep no more. Early mornings are their worst time, and by evenings the blues may have receded a little.

These diurnal swings of mood are characteristic. Physical symptoms of vague pains, headaches, backache, and palpitations, and often a fear of cancer, may dominate their lives, adding to the mental miseries. Feelings of guilt, wholly inappropriate, are mixed with a sense of inadequacy; they blame themselves for family misfortunes and sometimes for the evils of the world. Spells of restlessness and agitation may colour the picture. Medical attention is needed early in depression. Suicide can occur, but is rare in Parkinson's disease. Symptoms respond well to antidepressant drugs of the tricyclic group given for 6 to 12 months, sometimes longer. Results are generally very good. There is clear evidence that depression contributes a substantial element to the cognitive impairment of the disease. Its cause remains debatable, but there is little doubt that organic factors are crucial to its genesis.

Confusion and hallucinations

Both in younger patients and in the early stages of the disease these symptoms are uncommon. Many people over the age of seventy have periods of memory lapses, disorientation, and confusion. Deafness and impaired vision can lead to hallucinations in non-parkinsonian subjects. When they occur in Parkinson's disease they may be the result of aging effects alone, or they may be caused by anti-parkinsonian drugs of all types. Symptoms may at first be intermittent, and more noticeable at night and in strange surroundings, such as hospitals or nursing homes. Disorientation may be related to time, place, or person. The patient is bewildered and does not know where she or he is, nor what time of day it is. Recent information is imperfectly registered, so that she or he may deny having had lunch an hour ago, or forget having seen a recent visitor. Visual hallucinations often evoke people's faces, insects, or animals. Auditory hallucinations are less common, but fragments of overheard conversation or voices in a nearby room may be heard—with or without insight into the illusory nature of the experience.

Confusion may betray itself in disordered conversation or peculiar behaviour. Patients can pour milk into the teapot, put on clothes back to front, attempt to eat puddings with a knife, or find themselves unable to tie a knot in their tie or to use a comb or razor. These are varieties of dyspraxia often mistakenly called confusion. Victims may wander off and get lost.

Although these symptoms may occur in demented patients, where they are often not totally curable, they may just be a sign of sensitivity to drugs or evidence of an intercurrent infection, incipient renal or cardiac failure, or a reaction to surgery or anaesthesia. They may necessitate reduction in antiparkinsonian medication, and thereby cause increasing physical dependency. But it is easier to handle a sane but physically slow patient than a more mobile confused one.

When a parkinsonian patient first shows signs of confusion the first suspicion should be that it is induced by one or more components of his medication. Reduction or cessation of the offending drug may allow the return to sanity. In the elderly, in who so many other factors that can cause this state are so common, it may be prudent to withdraw all drug therapies, under careful observation. If the mental disorder continues when all other causes have been eliminated, it is likely that the basis lies in the Parkinson's disease itself, with the associated dementia or cortical Lewy-body disease.

Cognitive disorders

A variety of neurobehavioural changes and cognitive disorders have been shown in a high proportion of non-demented subjects with Parkinson's disease. They include disorders of memory, visuo-spatial function, and speed of central processing in both motor and psychological areas. This last is often called 'bradyphrenia', and has been related to frontal lobe dysfunction.

One view is to regard these disorders as precursors of dementia which occurs in between 10 and 30 per cent of patients. Follow-up studies to establish this hypothesis are not yet available. Thus, the possibility of their being selective functional disorders, independent of parkinsonian dementia, remains.

Refined neuro-psychological tests have disclosed a bewildering battery of abnormality.[2-5] Impairments of word fluency, memory scanning, sustained attention, and event-related potentials have been shown. Brown and Marsden[6] postulated an uncoupling or slowing of reaction times which produces a global slowing in the setting of perceptual–motor responses. There are also frequent reductions in planning motor sequences, in selective focused attention, in the ability to change mental and motor 'sets', and in problem solving. These are held to be frontal[7] or prefrontal in origin. Prefrontal disorders tested have shown defects in planning, switching or attention shifting, abstract thinking, concept building, and formation of models of the outside world. Abnormalities have also been shown in episodic learning and in specifically-directed search in remote memory for lexical, semantic, and autobiographical content. Psychologists have tried to erect models or paradigms of specific prefrontal defects and to match them with defects in Parkinson's disease patients. The tests unfortunately are riddled with uncertainties of both sensitivity and specificity. A recent exhaustive review concludes that 'we found little to bear out the claim of frontal involvement'. But the last word on this aspect is yet to be heard.

It is of interest that levodopa improves motor problems in almost all cases, but has little consistent effect in cognitive tasks, apart from an enhanced alertness and drive in some subjects. The frequency of depression[8] has led some to interpret these protean phenomena as subtle consequences of depression; others have argued the converse: that depression may be the result of slowed organic cognitive processing.

Dementia

Dementia implies an organically-caused decline in intellect, memory, and the ability to make rational decisions and judgements. It is a common threat to Parkinson's disease patients.[9] This has, without doubt, been overemphasized. Many parkinsonian patients are not affected in this way and never become demented. In later life both Parkinson's disease and Alzheimer's disease, the most frequent cause of dementia, are common. At the age of seventy, about 5 to 10 per cent of the non-parkinsonian population show some signs of dementia, and over half of these will be suffering from Alzheimer's disease.[10] Thus there is a chance that some patients, purely by coincidence, have both parkinsonism and dementia. The patient with Parkinson's disease has no greater chance than anybody else of having Alzheimer's disease— if both diseases are stringently defined. But the combination of both diseases markedly impairs the outlook. If the dementing illness is apparent at the onset of Parkinson's disease, the physician should suspect diffuse or cortical Lewy-body disease, and the prognosis is bad. If such patients are given levodopa drugs for their parkinsonian symptoms, they can tolerate only small doses, and are notably prone to side-effects, particularly confusional states and hallucinations. In other words, dementia limits the amount of levodopa it is possible to give, and the control of parkinsonian symptoms is less satisfactory for this reason. Families will need all the welfare services possible to cope with the patient at home. Ultimately periods in longer term hospitals or private nursing homes may be necessary.

Criteria

Precise delineation of these two overlapping syndromes is difficult. Criteria for dementia are controversial. 'Global intellectual failure', 'non-specific behavioural incompetence referrable to brain disease' (Benton and Sivan), and 'organic brain syndrome' are but a few of the offerings in an unsatisfactory literature.

DSM-III criteria are:

(1) loss of intellectual abilities of such severity as to interfere with social or occupational functioning;

(2) memory impairment;

(3) at least one of the following:
    (a) impairment of abstract thinking,
    (b) impaired judgement,
    (c) other disturbance of higher cortical function,
    (d) personality change;

(4) state of consciousness not clouded;

(5) either:
    (a) evidence . . . of a specific organic factor . . . aetiologically relevant . . . or
    (b) an organic factor . . . can be presumed if conditions other than organic mental disorders have been reasonably excluded and if the behavioural change represents cognitive impairment in a variety of areas.

Differential diagnosis of dementia in Parkinson's disease

In the patient suffering from Parkinson's disease motor disabilities make assessment of social competence very difficult, and thus hamper the application of some of these criteria. Differential diagnosis of the cause of dementia is also problematical and reversible causes must always be excluded. It is a tragedy if infective and metabolic causes, as well as subdural haematomata, benign tumours, or communicating hydro-cephalus, are overlooked—at any age. Toxi-confusional states (see p. 65–6) are an ever-present and potentially reversible diagnostic trap. Depressive pseudo-dementia is another potential pitfall, especially since depression is so common in Parkinson's disease, with cited estimates of prevalence varying between 20 and 90 per cent. Since extrapyramidal signs[11] indistinguishable from mild Parkinson's disease occur in at least 30 per cent of patients suffering from primary Alzheimer's disease, this too can be a source of misdiagnosis. Meticulous clinical assessment and neurocognitive tests and investigations, often including CT or MRI, are necessary to avoid a diagnostic error which probably occurs in 25 per cent of subjects.

Despite this, estimates suggest an incidence of between 20 and 81 per cent; but this is obviously a wide range of variation. The means of assessment is critical. Some errors lie in the mistaken diagnosis of Parkinson's disease in cases of drug-induced syndromes, and especially in arterio-sclerotic pseudo-parkinsonism and a variety of neuronal degenerations. The unmodified Folstein mini-mental-state examination alone can be misleading with false-positive or borderline results. Combined with selected non-verbal tests[12] it is improved; but a detailed interview with friends, relatives, and employers is crucial, and may avert diagnostic errors. Brown and Marsden have provided a just criticism of the varied criteria used in many of the studies[9] which explains their wide variation. Better surveys have been based on samples of an entire community; figures of 20 to 40 per cent have been obtained in four such studies.

Dementia and Lewy-body disease

Pathological studies have failed to show convincing Alzheimer's disease changes in a significantly increased degree in the brains of Parkinson's disease patients. Diffuse Lewy-body disease describes the presence of eosinophillic hyaline inclusions in both subcortical and cortical areas. The relationship of localized 'brain-stem Lewy-body disease' with Parkinson's disease is accepted. Cortical Lewy-bodies are uncommon in uncomplicated Parkinson's disease. The use of anti-ubiquitin immuno-cytochemistry has shown[13] that the severity of dementia is related to quantitatively measured Lewy-body density in the cortex, whilst subcortical components make a much less significant contribution. Diffuse Lewy-body disease appears to be present in unselected cases of dementia with a frequency varying from 5 per cent to almost 25 per cent. The clinical correlates in Parkinson's disease are dementia with aphasia, agnosia, and apraxia, and since the Lewy-bodies are found in up to 4 per cent of all cortical neurons, and in a much higher percentage in deeper cortical neurons, they probably contribute directly to the fall-out of neuronal function leading to dementia. Their mode of genesis is, however, uncertain, and they may simply be the hallmarks of the more fundamental process which causes the neurons to die.

   Current thinking favours the presence of cortical Lewy-body disease as the basis for dementia in Parkinson's disease. The role of the common cholinergic depletion founded on degeneration of Meynert's basal nucleus and its ascending cholinergic pathway remains uncertain. Senile plaques are common in Parkinson's disease patients, but are non-specific and not a reliable index of Alzheimer's disease unless quantitative studies are performed in which neurofibrillary tangles, granulovacuolar degeneration of the hippocampus, and Hirano bodies can be demonstrated.

References

1. Eatough, V. M., Kempster, P., Lees, A. J., and Stern, G. M. (1989). Pre-morbid personality in Parkinson's disease. In *Parkinson's*

disease, (ed. M. Streiffler), Advances in Neurology. Raven Press, New York. [Cited by A. J. Lees in *Parkinson's disease*, (ed. G. Stern), p. 409. Chapman and Hall, London, 1989.]

2. Flowers, K. A., Pearce, I., and Pearce, J. M. S. (1984). Recognition memory in Parkinson's disease. *Journal of Neurology, Neurosurgery, and Psychiatry*, **47**, 180–4.

3. Brown, R. G. and Marsden, C. D. (1988). An investigation of the phenomenon of 'set' in Parkinson's disease. *Movement Disorders*, **3**, 152–61.

4. Stern, Y., Mayeux, R., Rosen, J., and Ilson, J. (1983). Perceptual motor dysfunction in Parkinson's disease: a deficit in sequential and predictive voluntary movement. *Journal of Neurology, Neurosurgery, and Psychiatry*, **46**, 145–51.

5. Sagar, H. J., Sullivan, E. V., Gabrielli, J. D. E., *et al.* (1988). Temporal ordering deficits and bradyphrenia in Parkinson's disease. *Brain*, **111**, 525–39.

6. Brown, R. G. and Marsden, C. D. (1986). Visuospatial function in Parkinson's disease. *Brain*, **109**, 987–1002.

7. Stuss, D. T. and Benson, D. F. (1986). *The frontal lobes.* Raven Press, New York.

8. Rogers, D., Lees, A. J., Smith, E., *et al.* (1987). Bradyphrenia in Parkinson's disease and psychomotor retardation in depressive illness: an experimental study. *Brain*, **110**, 761–76.

9. Brown, R. G. and Marsden, C. D. (1984). How common is dementia in Parkinson's disease? *Lancet*, **ii**, 1262–5.

10. Pearce, J. M. S. (1987). *Dementia: clinical aspects.* Blackwell Scientific Publications, Oxford.

11. Pearce, J. M. S. (1974). The extrapyramidal disorder of Alzheimer's disease. *European Neurology*, **12**, 94–103.

12. Pearce, J. M. S. (1987). Dementia. *Medicine International*, **47**, 1956–60.

13. Lennox, G., Lowe, J., Landon, M. *et al.* (1989). Diffuse Lewy body disease: correlative neuropathology using anti-ubiquitin immuno-cytochemistry. *Journal of Neurology, Neurosurgery, and Psychiatry*, **52**, 1236–47.

8 Clinical scales and monitoring

The need to provide objective measures of a variety of phenomena in the disease was prompted by the development of controlled clinical trials of drugs. Commendably obsessional neurologists were also attracted to the possibilities of providing measurable data for clinical comparisons.

Computerization has refined current procedures, both in execution and in recording. Mechanical and electronic gadgets are now available for quantifying tremor, bradykinesia, and gait. They tend to be elaborate, expensive, and time-consuming. Pegboard tests and the author's simpler match test require a count of the number of objects placed correctly in a unit of time: a measure of timed motor performance. Functional disability scales portray the daily problems of patients. Video recordings can be used to illustrate a patient's physical signs and response to clinical tests. Rating scales of various signs and disabilities, physical and cognitive, are freely available and user-friendly.

Purpose of Parkinson's disease scales and monitoring

The purpose is

(1) to summarize the salient symptoms, signs, and disabilities at any stage of the illness;

(2) to provide a reliable basis for comparisons;
    (a) in the rate of change of individual symptoms and signs,
    (b) in checking the overall change by total scores,
    (c) in monitoring responses to treatment, and
    (d) as a necessary ingredient in therapeutic trials of drugs, surgery, physiotherapy, speech therapy, or non-medical procedures (for example, naturopathy, acupuncture, homeopathy).

(3) Specific scales can be valuable to provide an objective assessment of the important non-motor difficulties. These embrace self-sufficiency and its opposite, disability; they indicate breakdown of the individual's ability to function independently. They are often called 'activities of daily living (ADL)'.

Problems in assessment

The intrinsic variation in the symptoms and signs may produce differing results in the same patient when tested a few minutes or hours apart.

Drug-induced fluctuations are also a great source of potential error. Tests should be performed at the same time each day, and more importantly, *at the same interval after the dose of drug(s) is given* (in the 'on' or 'off' state). Stress and diet may also confound attempts at measuring a stable situation.

Social disabilities may be differently represented by patient, spouse, and family; information from all of them may provide a truer picture.

Many scales are based on 'absent', 'mild', 'moderate', or 'severe' appraisals. These are subjective, and inter-observer error compounds the difficulties. The Webster score has specific criteria for each item, and goes some way to solving this problem, though inter-observer errors, of, say, 1 for each item, might in theory produce a 30 per cent error for the total. In some respects, the more crude the criteria (for example, in Hoehn and Yahr, see below), the less the margin for subjective error.

Dyskinesia scales are used to observe the type, extent, severity, and distribution of drug-induced movements. They must be related to time of day and to the time of each dose if significant fluctuations are to be observed, and if dose and timing are thereby to be adjusted with benefit. Psychological appraisal is also necessary in many patients, particularly in advancing disease, and if affective disorders, toxi-confusional states, cognitive impairments, or frank dementia are suspected or evident. For clinical purposes frequent, skilled observations documented by experienced medical and nursing staff are important, supplemented by one of the mini-mental tests that should be employed.

Stage, disability, and severity

We have several scales for classifying the stages of the illness. Overall severity is rated on the well-established, but probably over-simplified *Hoehn and Yahr* scale, shown below.

Hoehn and Yahr scale

Five stages have been arbitrarily assigned by Hoehn and Yahr[2]

Stage I	unilateral disease only
II	bilateral mild disease
III	bilateral disease with early impairment of postural stability
IV	severe disease requiring considerable assistance
V	confinement to bed or wheelchair unless aided

There is also a detailed schedule describing problems in walking, feeding, dressing, hygiene, and speech which comprises five items measured on a ten-point scale; this is the *North Western University Disability Scale:*

North Western University Disability Scale

Scale A: Walking

Never walks alone

  0 Cannot walk at all, even with maximum assistance.
  1 Needs considerable help even for short distances, cannot walk outdoors with help.
  2 Requires moderate help indoors; walks outdoors with considerable help.
  3 Requires potential help indoors and active help outdoors.

Sometimes walks alone

  4 Gropes from room to room without assistance; never walks alone outdoors.
  5 Only moderate difficulty indoors; occasionally walks outdoors without assistance.
  6 Walks short distances with ease; rarely walks long distances alone.

Always walks alone

  7 Very slow and shuffling gait; posture grossly affected; mild propulsion; turning is difficult.
  8 Quality of gait poor, rate slow; posture moderately affected.
  9 Gait and posture almost normal; turning is the most difficult task.
10 Normal.

Score in boxes ☐

Scale B: Dressing

Requires complete assistance

  0 Patient a hindrance rather than a help to assistant.
  1 Movements of patient neither help nor hinder assistant.
  2 Can give some help through bodily movements.
  3 Gives considerable help through bodily movements.

Requires partial assistance

  4 Performs only gross dressing activities alone (hat, coat).
  5 Performs about half of dressing activities independently.
  6 Performs more than half of dressing activities independently.
  7 Handles all dressing alone with the exception of fine activities (tie, and so on).

Complete self-help

  8 Dresses self completely with slowness and great effort.

9   Dresses self completely with only slightly more time and effort than normal.
10 Normal.

Scale C: Hygiene

Requires complete assistance

0   Unable to maintain proper hygiene even with maximum help.
1   Reasonable good hygiene maintained, but little help given to assistant.
2   Hygiene maintained well; give help to assistant.

Requires partial assistance

3   Performs a few tasks alone with assistant nearby.
4   Requires assistance for half of toilet needs.
5   Requires assistance for some tasks not difficult in terms of co-ordination.
6   Manages most of personal needs alone.

Complete self-help

7   Hygiene maintained independently, but with effort and slowness, accidents are not infrequent; may employ substitute methods.
8   Hygiene activities are moderately time-consuming; no substitute methods.
9   Hygiene maintained normally, slight slowness.
10 Normal.

Scale D: Eating and Feeding
(*Figure separately and add the two scores)

*Eating**

0   Eating is so impaired that a hospital setting is required.
1   Eats only liquids and soft foods—these are consumed very slowly.
2   Liquids and soft foods handled with ease; hard foods occasionally eaten.
3   Eats some hard foods routinely, but requires time and effort.
4   Follows a normal diet, chewing and swallowing laboured.
5   Normal.

*Feeding**

0   Requires complete assistance.
1   Performs only a few feeding tasks independently.
2   Performs most feeding activities alone, slowly and with effort; requires help with specific tasks (cutting meat, filling cup).
3   Handles all feeding alone with moderate slowness; still may get assistance in specific situations (cutting meat in restaurant).
4   Fully feeds self with rare accidents; slower than normal.
5   Normal.

Scale E: Speech

0   Does not vocalize at all.
1   Vocalizes but rarely for communicative purposes.

2 Vocalizes to call attention to self.
3 Attempts to use speech for communications, difficulty in initiation, may stop in middle of phrase and be unable to continue.
4 Uses speech for most communication; articulation unintelligible; occasional difficulty in initiation; speaks in single words or short phrases.
5 Speech always employed for communication, articulation still very poor; usually uses complete sentences.
6 Speech can always be understood if listener pays close attention.
7 Communication easy although speech impairment detracts from content.
8 Speech easily understood, but voice or speech rhythm may be distorted.
9 Speech entirely adequate—minor voice disturbances present.
10 Normal.

Total NW Score

The *Barthel index* is another useful but non-specific list of abilities in daily activities.

The *Schwab and England capacity for daily living scale* (see within the UPDRS scale, end of chapter) is a ten-point scoring system in which each 10 per cent increment has a specific definition (100 per cent indicates normal function, 0 per cent indicates total disability).

The *Webster scale* comprises 10 items graded 0–3 each, producing a maximum score of 30 (most severe). There are two additional features which may be useful: a check on balance, and the ability to get up from a chair. I also add dyskinesia, which can be amplified, and a note of the presence or absence of confusion, hallucinosis, and dementia. This scale takes 5–10 minutes to complete for an experienced observer, and since there are necessary and specific criteria for each item (not absent, mild, moderate, or severe) the error rate is small.

Webster Rating Scale

I. Bradykinesia of hands—including handwriting

0 No involvement.
1 Detectable slowness.
2 Moderate slowness.
3 Severe slowness. Unable to write or button clothes.

II. Rigidity

0 None detectable.
1 Mild rigidity detectable only on activation.
2 Moderate rigidity detectable at rest.
3 Severe resting rigidity.

III. Posture

0 Normal posture. Head flexed forward less than 4 inches.
1 Beginning poker spine. Head flexed forwards up to 5 inches.
2 One or both arms flexed but still below waist.
3 Simian posture.

IV. Upper extremity swing

0 Swings both arms well.
1 One arm definitely decreased in amount of swing.
2 One arm fails to swing.
3 Both arms fail to swing.

V. Gait

0 Steps out well with 18–30 inch stride. Turns effortlessly.
1 Stride 12–18 inch, strikes one heel, takes several steps to turn.
2 Stride 6–12 inch. Both heels strike floor forcefully.
3 Shuffling gait and/or propulsion and intermittent freezing.

VI. Tremor

0 No detectable tremor found.
1 Mild fine-amplitude tremor, may be asymptomatic.
2 Severe but constant, patient retains some control of hands.
3 Constant and severe. Writing and feeding are impossible.

VII. Facies

0 Normal. Full animation. No stare.
1 Detectable immobility.
2 Moderate immobility. Drooling may be present.
3 Frozen facies. Mouth open. Drooling may be severe.

VIII. Seborrhoea

0 None.
1 Increased perspiration. Secretion remains thin.
2 Obvious oiliness present. Secretion much thicker.
3 Marked seborrhoea, entire face and head covered by thick secretion.

IX. Speech

0 Clear, loud, resonant, easily understood.
1 Beginning of hoarseness with loss of inflection and resonance.
  Good volume and still easily understood.
2 Moderate hoarseness and weakness. Beginning of dysarthria, hesitancy,
  stuttering, difficult to understand.
3 Marked harshness and weakness. Very difficult to hear and understand.

X. Self-care

0 No impairment.
1 Still provides full self-care but rate of dressing definitely impeded. Able to
  live alone and often still employable.

2 Requires help in certain critical areas, such as turning in bed, rising from chairs, and so on. Very slow in performing most activities but manages by taking much time.
3 Continuously disabled. Unable to dress, feed himself, or walk alone.

Balance

0 Normal.
1 Abnormal, but recovers unaided.
2 Would fall if not caught by examiner.
3 Cannot stand steadily.

Arising from a chair

0 Normal.
1 Slow, needs to use arms.
2 May need several attempts, but can get up without help.
3 Unable to rise without help.

Total Webster Score

Webster score for Parkinson's disease—Summary

Bradykinesia of hands
Rigidity
Posture
Arm swing
Gait
Tremor
Facies
Seborrhoea
Speech
Self-care
Total   /30 date: time:

Additional items suggested (scored 0–3):

balance/rising from chair/dyskinesia
Mental state: confusion/hallucinosis/dementia

By repeated use of these scales it is possible to record individual physical signs and related problems and to measure the degree of improvement or deterioration resulting from any form of treatment. The *King's College Hospital scale* measures 13 clinical items and 6 disability components on a 0–3 scale. The *Columbia scale*, the *New York University scales*, the *Cornell University scales*, and later the *UCLA scales* were other comparable schemata designed to monitor responses to dopaminergic drugs during trials. The need for an agreed standardized scale was outstanding, and this led to the more recent *Unified Parkinson's Disease Rating Scale (UPDRS)* (see end of chapter) developed by Professor Stanley Fahn and colleagues.[1]

The Unified Parkinson's Disease Rating Scale (UPDRS)

This is the current response to the call for a standardized but comprehensive method of assessment, introduced in 1984 by Fahn *et al.* It comprises six sections rated 0 to 4 or 0 to 5 in different parameters. The first section describes intellect, thought disorder, depression, and motivation. The second rates 13 items of activities of daily living in the 'on' and 'off' phases. A motor examination is broken down into 14 aspects in section 3, which is based on the Columbia scale. Evaluations show good inter-observer concordance. Complications of therapy in the past week are shown in section 4, which includes dyskinesias, clinical fluctuations, and other complications. Observer agreement varies for this item. Section 5 is a modified *Hoehn and Yahr scale*[2] rated in 8 stages. Section 6 is the *Schwab and England activities of daily living scale.* The last two sections show the best inter-observer correlation. The scale as a whole is detached and objective, but time-consuming to administer.

Unified Parkinson's Disease Rating Scale, version 3.0—(February 1987) definitions of 0–4 scale
I Mentation, behaviour, and mood
1. Intellectual impairment:
    0 = None.
    1 = Mild. Consistent forgetfulness with partial recollection of events and no other difficulties.
    2 = Moderate memory loss, with disorientation and moderate difficulty handling complex problems. Mild but definite impairment of functions at home with need of occasional prompting.
    3 = Severe memory loss with disorientation for time and often place. Severe impairment in handling problems.
    4 = Severe memory loss with orientation preserved to person only. Unable to make judgements or solve problems. Requires much help with personal care. Cannot be left alone at all.
2. Thought disorder (due to dementia or drug intoxication):
    0 = None.
    1 = Vivid dreaming.
    2 = 'Benign' hallucinations with insight retained.
    3 = Occasional to frequent hallucinations or delusions; without insight; could interfere with daily activities.
    4 = Persisent hallucinations, delusions, or florid psychosis. Not able to care for self.
3. Depression:
    0 = Not present.
    1 = Periods of sadness or guilt greater than normal, never sustained for days or weeks.
    2 = Sustained depression (1 week or more)
    3 = Sustained depression with vegetative symptoms (insomnia, anorexia, weight loss, loss of interest).

4 = Sustained depression with vegetative symptoms and suicidal thoughts or intent.

4. Motivation/initiative:
0 = Normal.
1 = Less assertive than usual; more passive.
2 = Loss of initiative or disinterest in elective (non-routine) activities.
3 = Loss of initiative or disinterest in day-to-day (routine) activities.
4 = Withdrawn, complete loss of motivation.

II Activities of daily living (determine for 'on/off')
5. Speech:
0 = Normal.
1 = Mildly affected; no difficulty being understood.
2 = Moderately affected; sometimes asked to repeat statements.
3 = Severely affected; frequently asked to repeat statements.
4 = Unintelligible most of the time.

6. Salivation:
0 = Normal.
1 = Slight but definite excess of saliva in mouth; may have night-time drooling.
2 = Moderately excessive saliva; may have minimal drooling.
3 = Marked excess of saliva with some drooling.
4 = Marked drooling, requires constant tissue or handkerchief.

7. Swallowing:
0 = Normal.
1 = Rare choking.
2 = Occasional choking.
3 = Requires soft food.
4 = Requires NG tube or gastronomy feeding.

8. Handwriting:
0 = Normal.
1 = Slightly slow or small.
2 = Moderately slow or small; all words are legible.
3 = Severely affected; not all words are legible.
4 = The majority of words are not legible.

9. Cutting food and handling utensils:
0 = Normal.
1 = Somewhat slow and clumsy, but no help needed.
2 = Can cut most foods, although clumsy and slow; some help needed.
3 = Food must be cut by someone, but can still feed slowly.
4 = Needs to be fed.

10. Dressing:
0 = Normal.
1 = Somewhat slow, but no help needed.

2 = Occasional assistance with buttoning, getting arms in sleeves.
3 = Considerable help required, but can do some things alone.
4 = Helpless.

11. Hygiene:
   0 = Normal.
   1 = Somewhat slow, but no help needed.
   2 = Needs help to shower or bathe; or very slow in hygienic care.
   3 = Requires assistance for washing, brushing teeth, combing hair, going to bathroom.
   4 = Foley catheter or other mechanical aids.

12. Turning in bed and adjusting bed-clothes:
   0 = Normal.
   1 = Somewhat slow and clumsy, but no help needed.
   2 = Can turn alone or adjust sheets, but with great difficulty.
   3 = Can initiate, but not turn or adjust sheets alone.
   4 = Helpless.

13. Falling (unrelated to freezing):
   0 = None.
   1 = Rare falling.
   2 = Occasionally falls, less than once per day.
   3 = Falls on average of once daily.
   4 = Falls more than once daily.

14. Freezing when walking:
   0 = None.
   1 = Rare freezing when walking; may have start-hesitation.
   2 = Occasional freezing when walking.
   3 = Frequent freezing; occasionally falls from freezing.
   4 = Frequent falls from freezing.

15. Walking:
   0 = Normal.
   1 = Mild difficulty; may not swing arms or may tend to drag leg.
   2 = Moderate difficulty, but requires little or no assistance.
   3 = Severe disturbance of walking, requiring assistance.
   4 = Cannot walk at all, even with assistance.

16. Tremor:
   0 = Absent.
   1 = Slight and infrequently present.
   2 = Moderate; bothersome to patient.
   3 = Severe; interferes with many activities.
   4 = Marked; interferes with most activities.

17. Sensory complaints related to parkinsonism:
   0 = None.

    1 = Occasionally has numbness, tingling, or mild aching.
    2 = Frequently has numbness, tingling, or aching; not distressing.
    3 = Frequent painful sensations.
    4 = Excruciating pain.

III Motor examination

18. Speech:
    0 = Normal.
    1 = Slight loss of expression, diction and/or volume.
    2 = Monotone, slurred but understandable; moderately impaired.
    3 = Marked impairment, difficult to understand.
    4 = Unintelligible.

19. Facial expression
    0 = Normal.
    1 = Minimal hypomimia, could be normal 'poker face'.
    2 = Slight but definitely abnormal diminution of facial expression.
    3 = Moderate hypomimia; lips parted some of the time.
    4 = Masked or fixed facies with severe or complete loss of facial
        expression; lips parted $1/4$ inch or more.

20. Tremor at rest:
    0 = Absent.
    1 = Slight and infrequently present.
    2 = Mild in amplitude and persistent. Or moderate in amplitude but only
        intermittently present.
    3 = Moderate in amplitude and present most of the time.
    4 = Marked in amplitude and present most of the time.

21. Action or postural tremor of hands:
    0 = Absent.
    1 = Slight; present with action.
    2 = Moderate in amplitude, present with action.
    3 = Moderate in amplitude with posture holding as well as action.
    4 = Marked in amplitude; interferes with feeding.

22. Rigidity (judged on passive movement of major joints with patient
    relaxed in sitting position. Cogwheeling to be ignored):
    0 = Absent.
    1 = Slight or detectable only when activated by mirror or other
        movements.
    2 = Mild to moderate.
    3 = Marked, but full range of motion easily achieved.
    4 = Severe, range of motion achieved with difficulty.

23. Finger taps (patient taps thumb with index finger in rapid
    succession with widest amplitude possible, each hand separately):
    0 = Normal.

1 = Mild slowing and/or reduction in amplitude.
2 = Moderately impaired. Definite and early fatiguing. May have occasional arrests in movement.
3 = Severely impaired. Frequent hestiation in initiating movements or arrests in ongoing movement.
4 = Can barely perform the task.

24. Hand movements (patient opens and closes hands in rapid succession with widest amplitude possible, each hand separately):
0 = Normal.
1 = Mild slowing and/or reduction in amplitude.
2 = Moderately impaired. Definite and early fatiguing. May have occasional arrests in movement.
3 = Severely impaired. Frequent hesitation in initiating movements or arrests in ongoing movement.
4 = Can barely perform the task.

25. Rapid alternating movements of hands: (pronation–supination movements of hands, vertically or horizontally, with as large an amplitude as possible, both hands simultaneously):
0 = Normal.
1 = Mild slowing and/or reduction in amplitude.
2 = Moderately impaired. Definite and early fatiguing. May have occasional arrests in movement.
3 = Severely impaired. Frequent hesitation in initiating movements or arrests in ongoing movement.
4 = Can barely perform the task.

26. Leg agility (patient taps heel on ground in rapid succession, picking up entire leg. Amplitude should be about 3 inches):
0 = Normal.
1 = Mild slowing and/or reduction in amplitude.
2 = Moderately impaired. Definite and early fatiguing. May have occasional arrests in movement.
3 = Severely impaired. Frequent hesitation in initiating movements or arrests in ongoing movement.
4 = Can barely perform the task.

27. Arising from chair (patient attempts to rise from a straight-backed wood or metal chair, with arms folded across chest):
0 = Normal.
1 = Slow; or may need more than one attempt.
2 = Pushes self up from arms of seat.
3 = Tends to fall back and may have to try more than one time, but can get up without help.
4 = Unable to rise without help.

28. Posture:
    0 = Normal erect.
    1 = Not quiet erect, slightly stooped posture; could be normal for older
       person.
    2 = Moderately stooped posture, definitely abnormal; can be slightly
       leaning to one side.
    3 = Severely stooped posture with kyphosis; can be moderately leaning to
       one side.
    4 = Marked flexion with extreme abnormality of posture.

29. Gait:
    0 = Normal.
    1 = Walks slowly, may shuffle with short steps, but not festination or
       propulsion.
    2 = Walks with difficulty, but requires little or not assistance; may have
       some festination, short steps, or propulsion.
    3 = Severe disturbance of gait, requiring assistance.
    4 = Cannot walk at all, even with assistance.

30. Postural stability (response to sudden posterior displacement
    produced by pull on shoulders while patient erect with eyes open
    and feet slightly apart. Patient is prepared):
    0 = Normal.
    1 = Retropulsion, but recovers unaided.
    2 = Absence of postural response; would fall if not caught by examiner.
    3 = Very unstable, tends to lose balance spontaneously.
    4 = Unable to stand without assistance.

31. Body bradykinesia and hypokinesia (combining slowness
    hesitancy, decreased armswing, small amplitude, and poverty of
    movement in general):
    0 = None.
    1 = Minimal slowness, giving movement a deliberate character; could be
       normal for some persons. Possibly reduced amplitude.
    2 = Mild degree of slowness and poverty of movement which is definitely
       abnormal. Alternatively, some reduced amplitude.
    3 = Moderate slowness, poverty or small amplitude of movement.
    4 = Marked slowness, poverty or small amplitude of movement.

IV Complications of therapy (in the past week)
A Dyskinesias

32. Duration: What proportion of the waking day are dyskinesias
    present? (historical information):
    0 = None.
    1 = 1–25% of day.
    2 = 26–50% of day.

3 = 5–75% of day.
4 = 76–100% of day.

33. Disability: how disabling are the dyskinesias? (historical information; may be modified by office examination):
0 = Not disabling.
1 = Mildly disabling.
2 = Moderately disabling.
3 = Severely disabling.
4 = Completely disabled.

34. Painful dyskinesias: How painful are the dyskinesias?
0 = No painful dyskinesias.
1 = Slight.
2 = Moderate.
3 = Severe.
4 = Marked.

35. Presence of early-morning dystonia (historical information):
0 = No.
1 = Yes.

B   Clinical fluctuations

36. Are any 'off' periods predictable as to timing after a dose of medication?
0 = No.
1 = Yes.

37. Are any 'off' periods unpredictable as to timing after a dose of medication?
0 = No.
1 = Yes.

38. Do any of the 'off' periods come on suddenly (for example, over a few seconds)?
0 = No.
1 = Yes.

39. What proportion of the waking day is the patient 'off' on average?
0 = None.
1 = 1–25% of day.
2 = 26–50% of day.
3 = 51–75% of day.
4 = 76–100% of day.

C   Other complications

40. Does the patient have anorexia, nausea, or vomiting?
0 = No.
1 = Yes.

41. Does the patient have any sleep disturbances (for example, insomnia or hypersomnolence)?
    0 = No.
    1 = Yes.

42. Does the patient have symptomatic orthostatis?
    0 = No.
    1 = Yes.

Record the patient's blood pressure, pulse, and weight on the scoring form

V Modified Hoehn and Yahr staging

Stage 0   = No signs of disease.
Stage 1   = Unilateral disease.
Stage 1.5 = Unilateral plus axial involvement.
Stage 2   = Bilateral disease, without impairment of balance.
Stage 2.5 = Mild bilateral disease, with recovery on pull test.
Stage 3   = Mild to moderate bilateral disease; some postural instability; physically independent.
Stage 4   = Severe disability; still able to walk or stand unassisted.
Stage 5   = Wheelchair bound or bedridden unless aided.

VI Schwab and England activities of daily living scale

100% Completely independent. Able to do all chores without slowness, difficulty, or impairment. Essentially normal. Unaware of any difficulty.

90% Completely independent. Able to do all chores with some degree of slowness, difficulty, and impairment. Might take twice as long. Beginning to be aware of difficulty.

80% Completely independent in most chores. Takes twice as long. Conscious of difficulty and slowness.

70% Not completely independent. More difficulty with some chores. Three to four times as long in some. Must spend a large part of the day with chores.

60% Some dependency. Can do most chores, but exceedingly slowly and with much effort. Errors; some impossible.

50% More dependent. Help with half, slower, and so on. Difficulty with everything.

40% Very dependent. Can assist with all chores, but few alone.

30% With effort, now and then does a few chores alone or begins alone. Much help needed.

20% Nothing alone. Can be a slight help with some chores. Severe invalid.

10% Totally dependent, helpless, complete invalid.

0% Vegetative functions such as swallowing, bladder, and bowel functions are not functioning. Bedridden.

Dyskinesia

Dyskinesia is important as a source of embarrassment and disability, though patients are commonly less troubled by it than are relatives. Dyskinesia often accompanies 'on' periods of motor activity and independence. It may occur at peak dose, during the wearing-off stage, or in its most troublesome form at both times—the so-called 'biphasic dyskinesia'. It varies in severity from inconspicuous choreic or athetoid movements of the mouth, shoulders, foot, or hand to violent jactitations which will throw the victim from a chair to the floor. Their timing and relationship to dosage is vital if treatment is to be refined. Dyskinesia scales are valuable in this context.

Dyskinesia scales

A   Duration; the time when dyskinesia is present during waking hours (per cent of waking hours):
0 = None.
1 = 1–25.
2 = 26–50.
3 = 51–75.
4 = 76–100.

B   Severity of dyskinesia.
0 = noticeable, mild but not disabling.
1 = mildly disabling.
2 = moderately disabling.
3 = severely disabling.

Note: C. Additional scales can be made 0–3 for the degree of painful dyskinesia and for dystonias + / − pain.

Mental state

There are numerous full-scale mental state examinations and dementia scales, and a variety of short mental-function or mini-mental examinations. For the practising neurologist, to be of service they should cover the main aspects of cognitive function, orientation, memory, and ability to manipulate knowledge and visuo-spatial information, and also reflect both verbal and non-verbal functions. A detailed consideration is beyond the scope of this small book. Many favour the Folstein mini-mental-state examination.[3] Criticism has been mainly directed at the inadequate representation of right-hemisphere visuo–spatial performance. The author's modification[4] includes these aspects as an addendum and provides a total score out of 40 instead of out of 30. Its clinical utility has been validated in the wards and in clinics. Further refinements or alternatives will certainly be developed, but the assessment of the parkinsonian patient is inadequate without some such statement of their mental capacity.

Mini-mental-state examination (Pearce modification of Folstein)

Orientation

Score one point for each correct answer:
What is the time? . . . date? . . . day? . . . month? . . . year? . . .   5
What is the name of this ward? . . . hospital? . . . town? . . . county? . . .
country? . . .   5

Registration:

Examiner names 3 objects. Score up to 3 points for correct answers at first attempt. Use further attempts and prompting so that patient may recall items later.   3

Attention and calculation:

Ask patient to subtract 7 from 100, and then 7 from the result. Repeat this four times down to 65, scoring one point for each correct answer.   5

Recall:

Ask for the 3 objects in the registration test, scoring one for each.   3

Language:

Score one point for each of two objects named (pen/watch).   2
Score one point for correct repetition of this phrase: 'No ifs ands or buts'.   1
Score 3 if a 3-stage command is correctly executed or one for each stage, e.g.
'With the right index finger touch the tip of your nose, then your left ear'.   3
On a piece of paper write 'Close your eyes'. Ask the patient to obey:
score one point.   1
Ask the patient to write any short sentence with a subject and a verb.   1

Construction and spatial sense:

Draw a pair of intersecting pentagons; score one if this is correctly copied.   1

Additional test of right-hemisphere function:

Draw a triangle, a square, and a circle, OR construct three shapes with matches.   3
Draw a clock face, filling in the numbers. Take off one point for each error (two or more errors score zero).   2

Cross each of the lines shown inside the square (example in the centre); take
off one point for each omission.   5

| —   / | —   /   / | Albert's Test

        | —   / | —   /   / | Albert's Test

        —   / | | — | | /

        /   — | /   +   —   /   /

        / | /   \   — | | —

        —   /   — | | —   /   —

Total score 40

Conclusions

Rating scales are of considerable value, perhaps mostly in persuading
clinicians to examine the complex phenomena of both the disease and its
therapy. Intrinsic variations are prominent, and only by careful monitoring is optimal treatment likely to emerge from rational considerations of
the observed fluctuations. Scales are also an essential ingredient of
clinical trials, both medical and surgical. Skilled execution of the tests is
vital if meaningless data are to be avoided. Further refinements are
inevitable, but the choice of scales will depend on the time available, the
clinical setting, and the quality of staff charged with measuring the
varying phenomena. The UPDRS is undoubtedly the most comprehensive scale, but will occupy more time than is available to many
physicians. The Webster is a simpler test, easily applied both in busy out-
patient clinics and in the wards; it forfeits detail, but can be improved by
small additions such as those indicated above.

Videotaping has obvious advantages, but requires additional time,
staff, and storage space. Used with a set protocol it may provide the best
record for reference and comparison for the future. Its visual appeal is
self-evident.

References

1. Fahn, S., Elton, R. L., and members of the UPDRS development committee. (1987). Unified Parkinson's disease rating scale. In *Recent developments in Parkinson's disease.* (ed. S. Fahn, C. D. Marsden, M. Goldstein, and D. B. Calne), Vol. 2, pp. 153–63. Macmillan, New York.
2. Hoehn, M. M. and Yahr, M. D. (1967). Parkinsonism: onset, progression and mortality. *Neurology,* **17**, 427–42.
3. Folstein, M. F., Folstein, S. E., and McHugh, P. R. (1975). Mini-Mental State. A practical method for grading cognitive state of patients for the clinician. *Journal of Psychiatric Research,* **12**, 189–98.
4. Pearce, J. M. S. (1987). Dementia. *Medicine International,* **47**, 1956–60.

9 Treatment: general principles

From inability to let well alone: from too much zeal for the new and contempt for what is old; from putting knowledge before wisdom, science before art, and cleverness before common sense; from treating patients as cases, and from making the cure of the disease more grievous than the endurance of the same, Good Lord, deliver us.

Sir Robert Hutchison[1]

The principles of treatment are aimed at abolishing as far as possible the symptoms and disabilities caused by the malady. It is understood that no drugs yet available will actually modify the disease process nor, with the possible but unproven, exception of selegiline, will they affect its natural progression. What they will do is to improve or reverse symptoms by replacing some of the depleted essential chemicals necessary for neural transmission and normal movements. In general, most drugs used will either enhance dopaminergic transmission or impede cholinergic transmission (see Fig. 9.1). Our therapeutic limitations are considerable. Precise delivery of the right dose to counteract the constantly varying metabolic disorder is not possible. Nor can we deliver drugs solely to the affected areas of the brain. Further, we remain impotent in attempts to arrest the disease process and to shield the brain from the natural wages of normal aging and vascular disease.

The principal aims are:

1. Treatment should be tailor-made to suit the needs of each individual; it will need adjustments or fine tuning at intervals over the entire course of the illness. In Parkinson's disease it is not enough to put the patient on one tablet, three times per day, and leave it at that.

2. Treatment should always be governed by symptoms and by disability. Table 9.1 gives a rough plan of my usual practice; but there is much variation, and the roles of early selegiline and dopamine agonists have not yet been conclusively established. For example, at the onset, when symptoms may be very mild and inconspicuous, it is often best to give no drugs at all. In the end stages, it is often wise to reduce or withdraw drugs.

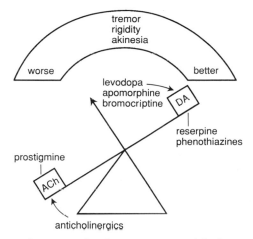

Fig. 9.1 See-saw schema of dopamine–acetylcholine imbalance in Parkinson's disease.

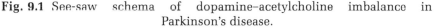

Table 9.1 Overall plan of disability linked with drug choices

Symptoms and disability	Treatment
no disability	no drugs ? selegiline
early tremor, slowness, symptoms a nuisance/embarrassment	anticholinergics (ACh), ? + selegiline ? dopamine agonist
good function but increasingly stiff or slow despite anticholinergics	amantadine +/− ACh, ? + selegiline
slow, marked tremor, falls; work or leisure difficult or in jeopardy	levodopa as Madopar/Sinemet +/− ACh ? + selegiline
late levodopa failure; wild fluctuations, dyskinesia	modify dose of levodopa, add bromocriptine, lysuride or pergolide
intractable fluctuations or 'on-off'	Madopar/Sinemet, add apomorphine s/c injections

Note. combinations are often used.

3. It is necessary to supervise the patient regularly to detect the right stage at which to begin or to alter treatment, and to detect and manage side-effects of drugs. Monitoring, by the serial recording of established clinical scales (see Chapter 8), improves records for purposes of comparison and trials.

4. Correct management means more than drugs alone. Active and positive efforts are necessary from the patient himself, and from relatives. Apathy and mental inertia are common features, doubtless due

to the primary disease process, but they are a therapeutic challenge; and the physician, for much of the illness, needs to persuade and to coerce the patient into making efforts to assert and maintain his independence as long as possible. Help is also needed from physiotherapists, occupational therapists, and various welfare services at certain times (see Chapter 14).

Patients should be referred to a specialist. Ideally, this should be at a neurological clinic. At the outset this serves both to confirm the diagnosis and to obtain advice about the immediate and future prospects of treatment. Often, the neurologist will arrange for regular follow-up at intervals which vary from two months to a year. General practitioners do not usually have the time or facilities necessary for the finer points required in initial diagnosis to separate the various causes of parkinsonism from idiopathic disease. Nor do they have the opportunities for the analysis of individual dose-related responses and fluctuations which is important in attaining optimal control and performance in each patient.

An outline of drug treatment

A rough outline of the various stages of the illness and the corresponding treatments available is shown in Tables 9.1 and 9.2.

Initial stages

In the asymptomatic patient, and in those with minimal tremor and rigidity and with slight slowness of movement, it is reasonable to withhold all drugs and to observe progress for as long as the symptoms and signs do not interfere with the sufferer's life and work. At this phase of the illness about 80 per cent of dopaminergic cells have been damaged, but the remaining cells increase their dopaminergic production and turnover, and release more dopamine at the striatal terminals.

The possible role of selegiline in delaying progression has to be confirmed (see pp. 93–4), but there is a case to be made for its early introduction at this stage.

Early disease

Once symptoms start to hamper work, dressing, feeding, or the pursuit of leisure activities, drugs should be started. We have referred earlier to the deficiency of essential dopamine in the brain, and to the excess of cholinergic transmitters relative to the deficiency of dopamine. Thus, early treatment consists of anti-cholinergic drugs (Table 9.2, and Chapter 10). Anticholinergics will secure modest improvements in tremor and rigidity. In small doses they produce few side-effects in younger subjects; but care is needed in the more elderly, who are at risk of glaucoma, prostatism, and toxi-confusional states as a result of these drugs.

There is current evidence (DATATOP trial; see below, p. 94) that selegiline given early will delay the time needed before the introduction of levodopa drugs. This may be purely by control of mild symptoms, but there is speculation (so far unproven) that selegiline may retard the advance of the disease.

Selegiline (1-deprenyl)

This is a weak antiparkinsonian drug; it may potentiate the effects of levodopa drugs, and it does reduce the 'on-off' swings, especially the immobile akinesia in the 'off' phase. It is well absorbed orally, reaching peak blood levels in 30 to 120 minutes. It is mainly metabolized in the liver. Its half-life is more than 24 hours, so that medication once a day is indicated. It blocks the presynaptic re-uptake of dopamine, hence increasing the dopamine available for the receptors. Its metabolites are amphetamine-like substances that have been shown independently to benefit parkinsonism.[2] There is an antidepressant effect which may be of additional benefit. A single dose of 5 mg or 10 mg each morning is well tolerated, and side-effects are not common.

Retarding progression of disease? Additional reason for the use of selegiline has been provided by the recent DATATOP (deprenyl and

Table 9.2 Some commonly-used drugs

Drug	Trade name	dose (mg)‡	dose (mg/day)
benzhexol	Artane	2 or 5	4–15
amantadine	Symmetrel	100	200
selegiline/ l-deprenyl	Eldepryl	5	5–10
Levodopa† + carbidopa	Sinemet†	50, 100, 250*	100–1000
bromocriptine	Parlodel	2.5, 5, 10	15–80

†Levodopa/benserazide (Madopar) is equivalent.
*Levodopa content only.
‡per tablet/capsule.

tocopherol antioxidant therapy of parkinsonism) trial.[3] This was based on the theory that free radicals and hydrogen peroxide released from degenerating neuronal proteins and neuromelanin produce toxic lipid peroxides. These cause dysfunction of cell membranes and ultimately damage the nigrostriatal pathway (see Chapter 3). The inhibition of MAOB and of oxidative pathways might therefore in theory retard such toxic damage and improve the prognosis. The DATATOP trial was based on 800 patients with early disease (stages 1 and 2, Hoehn and Yahr scale), aged 30 to 70, with a mean age of 61. Patients were not taking antiparkinsonian drugs or were able to withdraw from existing medication without deterioration. Depression and dementia were excluded. Deprenyl 10 mg/day, tocopherol 2000 IU/day, and placebo were used. The end-point was either the decision to treat with a levodopa drug or the elapse of 2 years; the trial was double blind.

At one year 176 controls and 97 deprenyl-treated patients had been deemed in need of levodopa: a 57 per cent reduction. Projected times for each group to reach the end-point were 15 months for controls and 26 months for the deprenyl group. The rate of clinical decline measured on standard scales and the risk of withdrawing from employment were both reduced by about 50 per cent in the treated group.

Possible explanations are firstly, a simple improvement of symptoms by the drug; secondly, a protective effect against some undisclosed environmental toxin damaging the nigral cells; and thirdly, a preventive effect on the decline to be expected in the established disease process. These results have yet to be confirmed: the end-point is to some extent subjective, but the implications are important. Impetus is added to early diagnosis, and to pre-clinical diagnosis, so that, if results are confirmed, the progression of the disease may be retarded or even halted. Many physicians now introduce selegiline in newly-diagnosed and early cases.

Amantadine

Later, amantadine may be introduced. This substance has mild dopamine-releasing properties and is weakly anticholinergic. It is a useful drug of mild-to-moderate potency (see Table 9.2), which may reduce tremor, rigidity, and bradykinesia. Toxicity is seldom a problem. Benefit may wane in about 50 per cent of patients after two or three months; if this happens, it is pointless to continue. After a year, some patients have swollen legs and livedo reticularis, but these are of cosmetic significance only, and not a manifestation of systemic illness caused by amantadine. The drug can be continued, and these side-effects disappear if the drug is stopped at a later stage. Within the first three years most patients need a levodopa drug.

Established disease

After about one to three years, many patients find symptoms are not adequately controlled by the above drugs. The judgement has to be made between non-disabling symptoms and signs of nuisance value, and those symptoms which significantly impede the patient and impair the quality of life or threaten employment. Once the sufferer is in the latter category, one of the levodopa drugs (see Chapter 11) is necessary, and should be slowly introduced (Table 9.2). When the latter is established with adequate benefit—usually within a matter of 6–8 weeks—an attempt should be made to withdraw slowly the anticholinergic medication, in the interests of simplicity; however, this is not always possible, since symptoms may increase as anticholinergics are withdrawn. If a combination of levodopa and anticholinergic is maintained, the dose of the latter should be kept to the minimum necessary, by trial and error. Anticholinergics have to be discontinued if cognitive function is impaired, if toxicity is unacceptable to the patient, and in older patients. Concurrent use of tricyclic antidepressants is often useful in countering depressive symptoms; these drugs have additional anticholinergic effects, with no significant interactions with established anti-parkinsonian agents.

Later disease: 'on–off' effects and dyskinesias

A variety of levodopa-induced side-effects tend to develop after one or two years of treatment in about half of all patients (see Chapter 11). Dopamine agonists, (bromocriptine, lisuride, pergolide, apomorphine) are introduced in some patients at this later stage. The indications are either that the levodopa drugs prove inadequate in controlling the parkinsonian symptoms, or that toxicity, 'on–off' fluctuations, or gross drug-induced dyskinesia prove refractory to fine adjustment of levodopa dosage and timing. If patients have psychotic symptoms on levodopa drugs, they are very likely to be worse on bromocriptine. Combinations of Madopar or Sinemet with a dopamine agonist may be valuable, and may permit reductions in the dosage of the levodopa drug. Details of drugs and regimes are amplified in succeeding chapters. An outline of the main drugs is shown in Table 9.2 (p. 93).

Mental disturbances

Mental disturbances may at any stage prove a barrier to successful treatment. Unwanted drug-induced effects include confusion, disorientation, and failing memory and concentration (see Chapter 6). They are part of the disease in some patients, partly caused by aging in others, and contributed to by all the major groups of antiparkinsonian drugs in varied degree. As the patient grows older abnormal movements or mental disturbances may make it necessary to reduce dosage. This usually produces a much calmer and more contented patient; but it is likely to increase the parkinsonian features—slowness and rigidity, difficulties in walking and posture, and falls. The stark choice sometimes amounts to a sane but immobile patient, or one who is mobile but plagued by hallucinations or psychosis. In the end, most families find it easier to handle the former and to accept that the patient is slow and perhaps immobile, but rational. Nursing may then be much easier for the family and helpers.

Some drug interactions and warnings

Certain drugs should not be used in parkinsonian patients. We have mentioned the major phenothiazine tranquillizers and antipsychotic drugs (neuroleptics). These drugs may also be suggested for nausea or dizzy attacks, but should not be used in Parkinson's disease. Monoamine-oxidase-A inhibitors used for depression are not allowed, but tricyclic antidepressants are in order. Patients with certain types of glaucoma or skin melanoma should not take levodopa (or anticholinergic drugs). Vitamin B6 (pyridoxine), present in multi-vitamin capsules and medicines, and used for premenstrual tension, can interfere with the action of levodopa (but not Madopar or Sinemet) and should be avoided.

References

1. Sir Robert Hutchison (1953). Modern treatment. Cited by Donald Hunter in Centerary of the birth of Robert Hutchison. *British Medical Journal*, 1971, **4**, 222–3.
2. Parkes, J. D., Tarsy, D., Marsden, C. D., *et al.* (1975). Amphetamines in the treatment of Parkinson's disease. *Journal of Neurology, Neurosurgery, and Psychiatry*, **38**, 232–7.
3. Shoulson, I. (1989). Deprenyl and tocopherol antioxidative therapy of Parkinsonism. *New England Journal of Medicine*, **321**, 1364–71.

10 Anticholinergic drugs

What drugs can make a withered palsy cease to shake?
—Tennyson, 'The Two Voices'

Deadly nightshade. (*Atropa belladonna*) is a solanaceous plant of hedgerows which was used in the nineteenth century as a source of belladonna alkaloids. They were used for sweating, colic, and as an ointment to dilate the pupils of young ladies who sought to enhance their beauty. Charcot and his pupil Ordenstein introduced belladonna in Parkinson's disease to control parasympathetic over-activity. Gowers used Indian hemp (*Cannabis sativa*), which also has anticholinergic properties, as well as being a possible dopamine re-uptake inhibitor.

Pharmacological action

The dopaminergic input in the nigrostriatal pathway inhibits acetylcholine-containing interneurons. Cholinergic neurons are also thought to mediate the effects of the dopaminergic neurons. Thus loss of inhibitory nerve supply increases the neuronal activity of cholinergic cells. This 'imbalance' results in a relative increase in cholinergic activity. Anticholinergic drugs act mainly by blocking postsynaptic muscarinic acetylcholine receptors. These receptors are sited in smooth muscle, cardiac muscle, and parasympathetic innervated glands, as well as in the brain.

Tremor and rigidity in experimental animals can be induced by cholinergic agents and blocked by atropine or scopalamine. In humans acetylcholine injected via a cannula into the globus pallidus increases contralateral tremor, which can be reduced by injection of an anti-cholinergic drug, oxyphenium. Duvoisin[1] showed that central stimu-lation with physostigmine, an anticholinesterase drug, increased parkinsonian signs in patients, and that these were reversed by anti-cholinergic agents. But peripherally-acting cholinergic agonists were ineffective in inducing or reversing signs. Some studies also suggest that they may inhibit the re-uptake of dopamine[2] into synaptic vesicles.

Clinical use and unwanted effects

Anticholinergic drugs are very useful for treating early tremor and rigidity, but are not as potent as levodopa in treating akinesia and bradykinesia and their attendant slowness, stooping, and falls. They are good at controlling salivation and drooling, but may cause a dry mouth. Patients with moderate or advanced disease are generally not controlled by anticholinergics, and require dopaminergic therapy. Efficacy is to some extent limited by the toxicity of full anticholinergic action on the pupil (paresis of accommodation), bowel (constipation), and bladder (retention), as well as by toxi-confusional states, psychosis, and impaired memory.

Their potency is significantly less than levodopa drugs or dopamine agonists. In early disease the overall score on rating scales is commonly improved by about 20 to 30 per cent.

Their potency is significantly less than levodopa drugs or dopamine agonists. In early disease the overall score on rating scales is commonly improved by about 20 to 30 per cent.

and any liability to glaucoma may be worsened and are relative contra-indications. Anticholinergics are particularly helpful in drug-induced parkinsonian states and in the now very rare post-encephalitic cases. It is doubtful if they actually potentiate levodopa drugs, or amantadine, though an additive effect may be useful. Similarly, it is not my experience that in patients with marked motor fluctuations caused by levodopa the use of anticholinergics prolongs clinical benefit, as has been claimed. Some workers have claimed that they are valuable in treatment of the dystonias accompanying chronic dopaminergic therapy. They are certainly effective in a proportion of patients suffering from the unrelated idiopathic torsion dystonia, but only when given in high dosage.

There is little to choose between the various drugs (Table 10.1) in terms of potency or side-effects.

Table 10.1 Common anticholinergic drugs

Drug	Trade name	Dose/tablet or capsule	Dose/day
Orphenadrine	Disipal	50 mg	100–300 mg
Benzhexol	Artane	2 or 5 mg	6–15 mg
Benztropine	Cogentin	2 mg	1–4 mg
Procyclidine	Kemadrin	5 mg	7.5–30 mg
Diphenhydramine	Benadryl	5 mg	5–10 mg

Classification

The drugs can be classified into three groups (Table 10.2). Choice should be determined by the physician's individual experience. **Antihistamines** causes sedation, though with orphenadrine this is not usually a problem. **Piperidines** are more potent; **benztropine** is probably the most potent, and has little significant sedative effect. In the UK, benzhexol and orphenadrine are the most commonly used drugs.

It should be remembered that other antiparkinsonian drugs may have significant anticholinergic properties. This is true of the tricyclic drugs (for example, imipramine, amitryptilene) often used with benefit in patients suffering from depression. Their actions are complex, and include enhancement of noradrenergic action, blocking re-uptake and probably storage of dopamine, as well as having significant anticholinergic effects on salivation and bowel and bladder function. Amantadine also has important anticholinergic properties.

Table 10.2 Classification of anticholinergic drugs

1. antihistamines:	orphenadrine (disipal); promethazine (phenergan); diphenhydramine (benadryl);
2. piperidines:	benzhexol (trihexylphenidyl, artane); procyclidine (kemadrin); biperiden (akineton).
3. tropines:	benztropine (cogentin).

Treatment

Treatment can start with one tablet twice daily (for example, benzhexol 2 mg, bd, or orphenadrine 50 mg, bd), or half of one tablet twice daily in the more elderly or infirm. Increases should be made every week (or two weeks in more elderly patients) until an adequate clinical improvement is apparent—usually within one to two months—or until side-effects occur. Patients are forewarned of unwanted effects, but many will tolerate minor degrees of constipation and a dry mouth, and these complaints may subside. Further adjustments of dose or timing enable patients to enjoy modest improvements in tremor and stiffness for a few years. Acquired tolerance is not a problem, but progression of the disease leads to an apparent loss of efficacy in many patients. The introduction of amantadine or dopaminergic agents is then necessary. Some patients, however, insist that anticholinergic drugs are beneficial for many years, and if cognitive impairment is not evident, and if the drug regime is not unduly complicated, the drug may be safely continued. The sudden withdrawal of anticholinergics must be avoided. It can, within two or three days, lead to a dramatic worsening, with rigidity, tremor, salivation, and immobility, not surprisingly accompanied by intense anxiety. When dopaminergic drugs are introduced, or when toxi-confusional or hallucinatory states or symptoms of dementia develop, the subject must be weaned from anticholinergics. Reductions are gradual, perhaps by one tablet every two or three weeks.

Amantadine

Amantadine, though not usually classed with the anticholinergic drugs, is included in this section because one of its several possible modes of action is as an anticholinergic agent. It was discovered in a remarkable fashion by that astute Bostonian neurologist, Bob Schwab:

'In early April 1968 a 58-year-old woman with moderately severe bilateral Parkinson's disease recounted to us that three months before, while taking amantadine hydrochloride 100 mg twice daily, to prevent the flu, she experienced a remarkable remission in her symptoms of rigidity, tremor and akinesia. These promptly returned on stopping the drug after six weeks. Her husband corroborated all of this.'

Schwab reported this as an example of serendipity.[3]

In Britain in 1969 the initial supplies of levodopa were irregular, and we took the opportunity[4] to assess the drug whose novel application had been discovered by Schwab. Its efficacy was quickly confirmed. Amantadine has significant antiparkinsonian effects, securing variable degrees of amelioration of tremor, rigidity, and akinesia. It is, however, less potent than the levodopa drugs. Its mechanism of action remains complex. It is anticholinergic, and enhances the synthesis of dopamine in the presynaptic storage vesicles and inhibits the re-uptake in the synaptic cleft. We observed a single case of facial dyskinesia induced by amantadine given without other drugs: clinical confirmation of its dopamine-mimetic properties.[5]

Peak plasma levels are reached after 2 to 8 hours, with a similar duration of clinical effect. Ninety per cent is excreted by the kidneys. The clinical application is the easiest and most trouble-free of all anti-parkinsonian drugs. Its benefits are apparent to patients within a few days. Dosage is standard, usually 100 mg bd, occasionally 100 mg tds. Further benefit does not accompany increasing dosage. Toxicity is minimal in the early stages, but the benefit wears off in a significant proportion of patients in the first two to three months. Others continue to show sustained and measurable improvement in motor performance as assessed on rating scales.

After one year some patients develop livedo reticularis, mostly on their legs; but this is harmless and slowly disappears if the drug is withdrawn for other reasons. Some patients develop dependent oedema, but investigation has shown this to be related to abnormalities in capillary circulation in the subcutaneous tissues, and it is not an indication of cardiac, liver, or renal failure. It too is reversible, and most patients can tolerate these side-effects, once reassured that they are benign. Amantadine has also been used in tardive dyskinesia, where it does not affect the psychiatric symptoms, and is thought to exert a protective effect on striatal dopamine receptors.

References

1. Duvoisin, R. C. (1967). Cholinergic–anticholinergic antagonism in Parkinsonism. *Archives of Neurology,* **17**, 124–36.
2. Coyle, J. T. and Snyder, S. H. (1969). Antiparkinsonian drugs: inhibition of dopamine uptake in the corpus striatum as a possible mechanism of action. *Science,* **166**, 899–901.
3. Schwab, R. S., England, A. C., Poskanzer, D. C., and Young, R. R. (1969). Amantadine in the treatment of Parkinson's disease. *Journal of the American Medical Association,* **208**, 1168–70.
4. Rao, N. S. and Pearce, J. M. S. (1971). Amantadine in Parkinsonism. *Practitioner,* **206**, 241–5.
5. Pearce, J. M. S. (1971). Mechanism of action of amantadine. *British Medical Journal,* **3**, 529.

11 Levodopa drugs

The revival of interest in Parkinson's disease in the late 1960s depended more on the clinical application of levodopa than on any other single discovery. Ehringer and Hornykiewicz had shown that dopamine and its metabolites were impressively depleted in the brains of patients.[1] The pioneering work of Cotzias,[2] almost single-handed, led to the clinical application, though the preparation was a crude D–L–isomeric mixture of dopa, which inflicted considerable toxicity on patients in the early stages of treatment.

In the UK, I remember being unable to persuade any pharmaceutical firm to obtain supplies in March 1967 when I had read Cotzias's paper; finally in the late summer of '67 I was able to obtain plastic bags of powdered D–L–dopa through the good offices of British Drug Houses, who somehow extracted supplies from Japan. My hospital pharmacy had to weigh 0.5 gm quanta into blank capsules; and, cautiously, I produced a special consent form for patients, (largely for my self-protection) long before ethics committees were invented.

Nonetheless, results were dramatic: a degree of improvement never seen before was observed within a few weeks of treatment.

Oliver Sacks later applied the term 'awakenings' to the new quality of life enjoyed by his patients, though many had post-encephalitic disease. Subsequent refinements found D–L–dopa discarded in favour of the purer, less toxic L-dopa (levodopa). Early optimism was justified by many trials showing sustained benefits for 90 per cent of patients.[3–6] We recognized that primary levodopa failures probably had some other form of parkinsonism, a suspicion confirmed by recent 'brain-bank' studies.

Levodopa is converted in the brain to active dopamine. The old pure levodopa preparation has now been replaced by combinations of levodopa with dopa-decarboxylase inhibitors (DDI), levodopa with carbidopa (Sinemet), and levodopa with benserazide (Madopar).

These drugs (Table 11.1) are the mainstay of drug treatment, and are more effective than other drugs presently available.

The striking benefits afforded by these drugs may in some cases slowly wear off after 5 to 10 years. But even at this stage, some patients retain some useful improvement. Individual needs and responses to therapy vary widely, so that the dosages or regimes mentioned here must be taken as guidelines.

Table 11.1 L-Dopa drugs

Drug	Trade name	dose/tab contents (mg)[1]	dose L-dopa/ day (mg)
levodopa with benserazide	Madopar[2] 62.5 Madopar 125 Madopar 250 Madopar CR	ld 50, benserazide 12.5 ld 100, benserazide 25 ld 200, benserazide 50 ld 100, benserazide 25	100–800
levodopa with carbidopa	Sinemet[3] LS Sinemet 110 Sinemet-Plus Sinemet 275 Sinemet CR	ld 50, carbidopa 12.5 ld 100, carbidopa 10 ld 100, carbidopa 25 ld 250, carbidopa 25 ld 200, carbidopa 50	100–800

1. ld = levodopa; 2. Madopar is the trade name of co-beneldopa; 3. Sinemet is the trade name of co-careldopa.

Levodopa drugs are the treatment of choice for moderate and severe Parkinson's disease. Rigidity, slowness, posture,[7] and often tremor are improved by levodopa drugs. Their good effects may be less marked in the elderly and in those with very long-standing illness, because dose-related toxicity may make patients unable to tolerate a dose large enough to control their symptoms.

Levodopa is best given as Sinemet or Madopar preparations, in which a dopa-decarboxylase inhibitor drug concentrates the levodopa in the brain and minimizes side-effects elsewhere in the body. For example, Sinemet 110 contains levodopa 100 mg, plus carbidopa 10 mg; and Madopar 250 contains levodopa 200 mg, plus benserazide 50 mg.

Clinical pharmacology

Dopamine itself does not cross the blood-brain barrier in appreciable quantities. By contrast, the precursors of dopamine, L-tyrosine and L-dihydroxyphenylalanine, easily cross the barrier. Tyrosine hydroxylase is the rate-limiting enzyme in dopamine synthesis, and its activity is greatly diminished in parkinsonian brains. Levodopa also crosses the blood–brain barrier and is converted to dopamine by decarboxylase enzymes, which are mainly located at the terminals of nigrostriatal neurons.[8] Dopamine exerts its antiparkinsonian effects at the dopamine receptor sites. Levodopa, however, has little affinity for the D_2 dopamine receptors.

Levodopa itself is a precursor of several metabolites, of which dopamine is the most important. Its absorption is good when given orally, with peak serum levels at 30 to 60 minutes. Absorption occurs in the duodenum and proximal small bowel via a saturatable transport mechanism for large neutral amino acids. Competition for absorption may arise from dietary amino acids, and has been shown to occur experimentally by reduction of levodopa absorption when methionine or L-tryptophan are administered at the same time. About half the dose of levodopa is decarboxylated by the enzymes in the first passage through the gut. The circulating level is approximately 30 per cent of an oral dose, but this increases to 60 to 90 per cent if levodopa is given with carbidopa.

High levels of gastric acid and large meals may slow gastric emptying and thus impede levodopa absorption. Serial blood estimations often show multiple peaks after a single dose, indicating erratic gastrointestinal absorption. These observations may explain in part the fluctuations[9] in performance so commonly observed (50 per cent of patients at 5 years) later in the disease. Typical values for plasma levodopa levels after oral Sinemet are:

time (hours)	0	1	2	4	8
plasma levodopa (ng/ml)	0	1700	1450	600	0

Clinical efficacy, seen as improvement in motor function, is extremely variable. In the newly treated patient, it lasts for about 4 to 6 hours after each dose, with a lag of 30 to 60 minutes after the dose before benefit is observable. Controlled release (CR) preparations provide lower peaks, usually of the order 700 to 1400 ng/ml, and persistent low levels of 300 to 800 ng/ml at 8 hours. This theoretically reduces the number of doses needed per day; but in practice small doses of CR preparations are used at roughly the same frequency, and larger doses (for example, 130–150 per cent) are necessary to try to achieve adequate peak clinical efficacy (see p. 114).

The advantages of the mixtures of levodopa with a dopa-decarboxylase inhibitor (DDI) are that the DDI reduces peripheral dopaminergic 'side-effects, enhances the speed of initial stabilization, and substantially reduces the early vomiting and syncope which attended treatment with pure levodopa. The effective dose of levodopa is reduced to about 20–25 per cent.

The drug is decarboxylated by dopamine-β-hydroxylase to dopamine, which in turn is decarboxylated at noradrenergic terminals to noradrenalin. Monoamine oxidases, notably catechol-O-methyl-transferase, are also an important metabolic breakdown pathway, producing oxidative and methylated metabolites. Dopamine is also formed in 5-HT cells by decarboxylation. Dopamine formation is followed by storage in vesicles in the presynaptic neurons and by release across the synaptic cleft to the postsynaptic receptor sites. Important re-uptake occurs at the synaptic cleft.

There is a greater loss of dopamine than of its oxidative metabolites in the disease, suggesting either that undamaged and functioning nigro-striatal neurons are adapting by increasing dopamine synthesis or increasing release in the storage vesicles. A related issue is whether the long-term administration of levodopa can contribute to the continuing degeneration of nigrostriatal neurons. This concept is of more than theoretical importance; if chronic dopaminergic drive hastens degeneration in dopaminergic neurons or in the receptors, it would be prudent to delay the inauguration of therapy as long as possible and to keep dosage down to the minimum necessary for satisfactory, but not perfect, control of symptoms. Clinical trials have so far provided no evidence, and many workers ignore this possible detriment, and strive for optimal treatment of symptoms from an early stage. This theoretical aggravation of the degenerative process is not supported by experimental work on mice; but species variation in susceptibility to extrinsic toxins and drugs—such as is seen in MPTP in rodents and primates—cautions against too ready extrapolation of these results to man. There is some evidence that chronically denervated receptors may sprout additional terminals and show increased sensitivity to transmitted dopamine. This has long been the explanation affirmed for the 'denervation supersensitivity' which is thought to be the basis of drug-induced dyskinesia (see Chapters 3 and 6), and also the tardive dyskinesia of chronic dopamine blockade resulting from neuroleptic drugs.

Introducing levodopa drugs

The indications for starting therapy with a levodopa drug have been discussed in Chapter 9. The principal stimulus is an inadequate response to anticholinergics and amantadine, evident in continuing and increasing symptoms, and the threat of disability in the home or at work. Treatment is started with a small dose (Madopar 62.5 or Sinemet 50 LS), taken once or twice daily with food (Table 11.1, p. 103). Smaller doses are used in the elderly.

All Madopar preparations are based on a 4:1 ratio of levodopa: benserazide. Sinemet 110 is based on a 10:1 ratio of levodopa:carbidopa; Sinemet plus is 4:1, and Sinemet CR is 4:1. In theory, it requires about 75 mg of dopa-carboxylase inhibitor (benserazide or carbidopa) to achieve full peripheral decarboxylation, and thus to concentrate the levodopa in the brain with minimal peripheral dopaminergic side-effects.

The dose is gradually increased, perhaps by 50 mg levodopa every 4 to 7 days, depending on age, length of history, mental impairment, and the individual's response. When the smallest dose necessary to produce acceptable control of symptoms and disability is reached the dose is deemed optimal—at that time. The initial response is usually clinically impressive. In the untreated patient with obvious bradykinesia, postural flexion, rigidity, and immobile features the results can sometimes be dramatic. The individual signs melt away within the first few weeks, and a slow, stooped, shaky wreck is transformed into a mobile, quickly moving, erect human being. Sadly, this does not always happen; and the milder the signs, the less dramatic the response. Tremor may be the most refractory symptom. It is good therapeutics to try to wean patients from other antiparkinsonian drugs when they have been satisfactorily stabilized on levodopa drugs. There is currently a case to be made out for continuing selegiline in the early years, for its potential action in impeding disease progression.

The best dose is often a compromise between near-total control of all symptoms and avoidance of side-effects. Many physicians like to keep a little in reserve for future needs. Most patients are untroubled by early side-effects, though occasionally nausea, vomiting, or fainting are a nuisance; but these are easily overcome by dose adjustments and timing. I prefer not to complicate therapy by adding other drugs such as domperidone or metoclopramide to counteract transient sickness.

As the disease progresses, the smooth effect and benefit throughout the day diminishes. Wearing-off occurs at the end of a dose, after three or four hours, when the patient is slow and rigid again. Or else the effects achieved are only partial, and the parkinsonian symptoms are incompletely controlled. The dose may then be increased to Madopar 250 tds or Sinemet 275 tds. Some patients may require four or, rarely, more doses per 24 hours. The increase will at first provide added potency and clinical benefit and longer duration of effect. But later these benefits may wane, or drug-related side-effects may emerge.

Wearing-off effect

After two or more years, the duration of action seems shorter. Wearing-off may be noted at the end of each dose (end of dose akinesia), before the next tablets are due (Fig. 11.1); or wearing-off may be noted on waking each morning (early morning akinesia) because the last evening's dose has worn off. Another common pattern reported by patients is a good response to morning doses, but poor or absent response in the afternoon or evening. Frankel et al.[10] have studied this phenomenon and shown that, if dietary factors attributed to lunch are eliminated, the levodopa levels in the plasma are similar at all times of day, the magnitude and duration of clinical responses are not different, and the

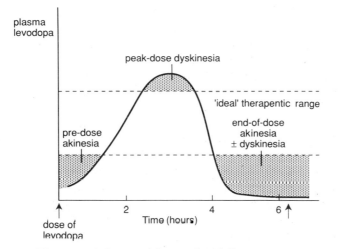

Fig. 11.1 Schema of dose-related fluctuations.

falling levodopa levels at which 'wearing off' symptoms occur are also similar after morning or afternoon doses. Slowness, stiffness, freezing, and falls are the most troublesome features. This stage is due to progressive reduction in the capacity of striatal cells to synthesize, re-uptake and store dopamine. This has been demonstrated experimentally in lesioned rats and confirmed in man by PET scans which show reduced storage and metabolites of administered [18F]6-fluorodopa. Confirmation is evident in the ability of patients in the 'off' phase to respond both to exogenous levodopa and to apomorphine. Thus the receptors retain the ability to respond to dopamine, but are deprived of their dopamine supply.

The natural history has been discussed in Chapter 4. The wearing-off effect is itself a sign of proceeding degeneration, being an indication of the changing pharmacokinetics and of the responsiveness of the dopaminergic receptor sites. It may be hard to distinguish progressing disease from the waning benefit of levodopa therapy. Shaw, Lees, and Stern[11] showed that after six years treatment, only 37 of 125 patients maintained their initial level of improvement, compared to 69 patients at two years after therapy. However, at six years 47 were still better than before treatment. Wearing-off had occurred in 65 per cent of patients, and unpredictable fluctuations (see pp. 112–15) in 10 per cent.

Psychiatric symptoms

Increasing age, a previous history of depression, underlying dementia, concurrent polypharmacy, and cerebrovascular incidents all predispose to mental side-effects of all classes of drugs used in the disease. Levodopa may cause early restlessness at night, vivid dreams, and sometimes nightmares and myoclonic jerks in the twilight state. Toxi-confusional states and visual hallucinations occur rarely in younger fit patients at the onset of therapy. Insight is often preserved, so that although the sufferers truly see the objects of their hallucinosis, they will later relate that they know they were unreal. Delusions may occur less commonly, and altered sleep–wake cycles may disrupt the family's equanimity. Aggressive behaviour is rare, but depression may be aggravated, though it may also improve *pari passu* with the increased physical freedom permitted by the drug. Many of these psychiatric symptoms are dose-related, and sedulous attention to attenuation of dosage may abolish them, with only minor reduction in efficacy. In older subjects, if toxicity occurs on tiny doses, it may eventually cause the physician to stop the treatment. Chronic confusional states may be mistaken for dementia—an error which has obvious therapeutic implications, since the former state may be in large part reversible. The suspicion that chronic levodopa therapy may actually cause dementia is unproven. After six years treatment with levodopa Shaw, Lees, and Stern found dementia in 32 per cent of patients, although more recent studies suggest a much smaller incidence, of the order of 10 to 20 per cent.

Drug-induced dyskinesia and dystonia

After one or two years, some patients develop abnormal twitching (choreic), dystonic, or writhing (athetoid) movements called 'drug-induced dyskinesia'. They typically occur 1 to 3 hours after a dose, when brain levels of dopamine are at their peak (Fig. 11.1). The movements affect the mouth, tongue, lips, and cheeks (oro–buccal–lingual dyskinesia), with twisting, writhing, or darting motions; sucking, licking, swallowing, or protrusion of the lips and tongue occur in an irregular fashion. They may affect the neck, producing forward, backward, or lateral movements resembling spasmodic torticollis. Dyskinetic jerks, chorea, athetoid writhing, and dystonic postures may distort the limbs and trunk. Painful clawing of the toes and hands are signs of drug-induced dystonia, which may occur at peak dose or in the wearing-off stages.

Dyskinesias more often trouble the patients' husbands or wives than the patients themselves, for while they are embarrassing and unsightly they often coincide with periods of physical activity which are welcomed by the sufferer. But they can be disabling, forcing patients to sit or lie on the floor rather than be thrown violently from a chair. If severe, they can be reduced, or less often abolished, by smaller doses of the drugs, which may then need to be given more frequently. The patient with dyskinesia on Sinemet 275 three times a day may be relieved of it by Sinemet 110 in 5 or 6 doses at 2- to 3-hourly intervals.

'On-off' attacks

'On-off attacks' may develop later. The 'on' phase occurs at peak dose, and the patient is then mobile and independent, but often has abnormal dyskinetic movements. The 'off' phase consists of sudden freezing, with feet sticking to the floor, and immobility, sometimes with a feeling of fear and panic. Patients may suddenly switch from 'on' to 'off' and from 'off' to 'on', 'like flicking on a light switch'. This is disconcerting, and may be wrongly thought to be of nervous or pyschological origin.

    'On-off attacks' are highly complex (Fig. 11.2). Undoubtedly irregular storage, release, and re-uptake of dopamine play a role; but there is also evidence of altered absorption and handling of administered levodopa—the pharmacokinetic factor. The latter depends on variation in rates of

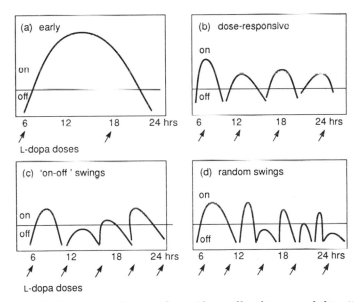

Fig. 11.2 (a) Early phase where 2 doses/day will achieve mobility ('on') for 24 hours. (b) Later dose-responsive fluctuations in performance on 4 doses/day. (c) Dose-related 'on-off' swings. (d) Random swings with frequent 'off' periods and random dyskinesias in 'on' phases.

gastric emptying, inefficient small-intestinal absorption, varying extra-cerebral metabolites of levodopa, and possible competition for transport across the blood–brain barrier by other large neutral amino acids. The improvement of function in the early morning, so commonly observed by patients, is called 'sleep benefit', but its mechanism is obscure. This long-recognized phenomenon of the restorative value of sleep was known to Shakespeare:

I'll strive, with troubled thoughts, to take a nap,
Lest leaden slumber peise* me down tomorrow,
When I should mount with wings of victory.

—(*Richard III* V. iii 105–7)

In Parkinson's disease sleep benefit is often ascribed to changes in dopamine receptor sensitivity and to natural circadian rhythms altering receptor or neuronal behaviour. The essential basis of the 'off' state is nigral cell loss and endogenous dopamine deficiency. The 'on' phase plainly depends on preserved function and sensitivity of dopamine receptors; indeed there is much to suggest a state of 'denervation hyper-sensitivity'. It has been suggested that the motor responses to both single-dose levodopa (as Sinemet 275) and apomorphine are of similar magnitude, and therefore that the principal factor in determining motor responsiveness is the presence of an intact postsynaptic receptor in the striatum.[12] However, the dose of apomorphine used in this study was 2 or 4 mg, and it is possible that higher doses might have produced a greater response as measured from the pre-dose 'off' motor score to the best score during the 'on' period. There remains much of these theoretical mechanisms which we do not yet understand. Patients can be dyskinetic in one limb and show Parkinsonian bradykinesia and tremor in another limb at the same time. Are there segmental divisions of motor function in the striatum showing different affinities or differing sensitivities to transmitted dopamine? Dyksinesia in the 'on' phase is most evident in the limbs most affected by parkinsonian signs. Dyskinesia is not readily induced in non-parkinsonian patients, but can occur in symptomatic parkinsonism due to multi-system atrophy. These clinical clues need further investigation; but to a large extent they are at present unexplained mysteries.

Smaller, more frequent doses may in part ease this difficult problem. These manipulations require patience and skill from both patient and physician. As time goes by the duration of benefit after each dose decreases; changing from, for example, Sinemet 275 tds to Sinemet 110 4 to 6 times a day may reduce dyskinesia and reduce 'on–off' attacks, but may also increase the duration and severity of parkinsonian slowness

*peise: to make heavy and so retard or weigh down.

and stiffness. Other strategies are tailored to the patient's needs. It is often helpful to give a larger dose early with breakfast; for example, Sinemet 2×110 to achieve greater mobility in the mornings. Patients who cannot get out of bed to the lavatory or who cannot turn over in bed may be helped by a small additional dose of Sinemet 50 or 100 mg levodopa at bedtime. Sleep confers marked benefit in some. If on rising they are mobile, and able to shave, bath and dress with reasonable speed, it may be prudent, for example, to postpone the first morning dose from 7 a.m. to 9 a.m., thus saving more treatment for later in the day, when it may be needed. It is often necessary to admit patients to hospital for a week or two for specialized care and frequent (hourly) checks and ratings of symptoms, side-effects, and dosage in order to achieve the fine tuning necessary for optimal performance. Assessments of neurological signs, neuro-psychological state, coincident or complicating general medical conditions, and cardiovascular, bladder, and bowel functions are carried out as required. This is often a sensible time to reappraise the problems and capabilities of the wife or husband and family and the adequacy of social support, housing needs, and appliances (see Chapter 14). It is often necessary to bolster the carers of the patient at home via community health resources and by liaison with the general practitioner, district nursing, and social services.

Side-effects of levodopa drugs

In addition to the pharmacological and dose-related fluctuations described, there is a wide variety of possible side-effects and toxicity due to levodopa drugs. They may affect many systems (Table 11.2). Their correction may require changes of dosage or timing, or the substitution of alternative preparations. It is generally inadvisable to prescribe one drug to counter the side-effects of another; for example, pressor drugs for faintness or antiemetics for nausea. The additional drugs so used may conceal important features, such as fainting as an indication of multi-system atrophy, or they may interfere with the primary treatment: for example, phenothiazines prescribed for nausea or anxiety will induce

Table 11.2 Side-effects of levodopa drugs

cardiovascular:	faintness, postural fall in blood pressure, arrhythmias.
cerebral:	vomiting, nightmares, hallucinosis, psychosis, dyskinesia, dystonia, and 'on–off' swings.
gastro-intestinal:	nausea, vomiting, anorexia.
miscellaneous:	increased libido, red urine, rashes.

dopamine blockade. Some patients may prefer Madopar to Sinemet and *vice versa*. Apparent side-effects may occasionally be abolished by a direct exchange of one for the other. In terms of general efficacy and toxicity the drugs are equal.[13] Minor differences in dosage (for example, Madopar 250 contains levodopa 200 mg, whereas Sinemet 275, the equivalent, contains levodopa 250 mg) and occasional idiosyncratic preferences may justify a change from one preparation to the other.

Fluctuations

In the early stages of treatment with levodopa compounds, a smooth even response throughout the day is obtained. This is apparent after the patient is stabilized on twice- or thrice-daily medication; the benefit extends beyond the pharmacological half-life, and is presumably due to repletion of neuronal dopamine stores and the steady release of dopamine from them. After one to three years fluctuations in motor performance often develop. These are evident in more than 50 per cent of patients after five years of treatment. They are related to the severity of the disease, the duration of the disease, and the duration of levodopa treatment. The mechanisms are not fully understood.[14,15] The main factors appear to be:

(1) loss of presynaptic receptor sensitivity to levodopa/dopamine;
(2) modification of post-synaptic receptor sensitivity;

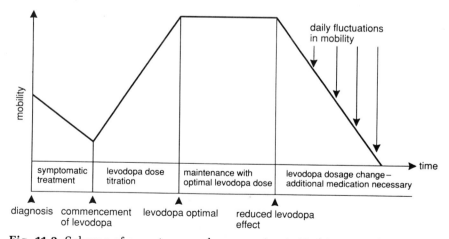

Fig. 11.3 Schema of symptoms and progression in Parkinsons's disease and the effects of levodopa.

(3) altered peripheral and central pharmacokinetics inhibit levodopa absorption from the G–I tract and its passage across the blood–brain barrier; and

(4) changes in non-dopaminergic neurotransmitter systems.

Clinical and pharmacokinetic tests have shown that continuous levodopa infusion by intraduodenal[16] or intravenous drip can eliminate much of the oscillation, and can override the 'off' stage. This shows that even late in the disease, the receptors are still in large measure responsive.[17]

Fluctuations in clinical phenomena

A number of regular clinical patterns of fluctuations in motor performance are seen. Their occurrence should be carefully noted and related if possible to the time of the previous and the next dose of medication. Many patients and their relatives can be inured to keeping a chart planned to show these effects, and are well able to do so. Notes should be made of:

1. End of dose wearing-off—4 hours after a dose.

2. Early morning wearing-off noted on waking.

3. Decreasing duration of 'on' phase to 1–3 hours after a dose.

4. Akinetic freezing and falls.

5. Peak-dose dyskinesia in 'on' phase 1–2 hours after a dose.

6. Painful dystonias, often end-of-dose or early morning.

7. Diphasic dyskinesia—1 hour after dose, then 1 to 2 hours later, before the next dose is due.

8. A variety of ballistic movements, stereotyped movements, myoclonus, and disturbances in behaviour which can occur.

If fine adjustments of the dose and timing of the levodopa drugs afford inadequate control, another group of drugs, the dopamine agonists, may be used. They stimulate the dopamine receptors, rather than supplying more dopamine. Bromocriptine (Parlodel), pergolide, and lysuride are the most used (Chapter 12). More recently, apomorphine has been found effective; but since this has to be given by regular injections, rather like the way a diabetic uses insulin, a trial of an oral dopamine agonist should be tried first (see Chapter 12). Selegiline, a weak antiparkinsonian drug, may occasionally in advancing disease be useful, in conjunction with Madopar or Sinemet in reducing the end-of-dose akinesia and the 'off' phases (see pp. 106, 109). Treatment with dopamine agonists is started with a small dose, taken with food. This is gradually increased until the smallest dose necessary to produce acceptable control of symptoms and disability is reached (see Chapter 12 and Table 11.1, p. 103 for the usual range of dosage).

Management of the refractory patient

This sad but common situation is characterized by:

(1) short periods of varying degrees of mobility and independence, punctuated by capricious episodes of

(2) akinetic immobility and freezing and falling in the 'off' stage.

(3) dyskinesia and dystonia of face, head, trunk, and limbs in the 'on' stage.

(4) an overall state of immobility for most of each day which is due to severe akinesia confining the sufferer to wheelchair or couch, but is punctuated by frequent falls, injuries, and dyskinetic periods of such violence that the patient has to lie on the floor or bed.

The difficulties are compounded by the fact that although in the early days these fluctuations have some predictability, being related to the time of the last dose of dopaminergic drug, later they appear at random. The patient's domestic and social life becomes chaotic.

There are several steps to be taken in order. **At first smaller doses** are used more frequently to avert higher peaks and troughs and their accompanying 'on–off' swings. Then, **the addition of selegiline** (if the patient is not already taking this drug) may reduce the 'off' periods; but the effect is seldom dramatic. The later **introduction of bromocriptine or lysuride** may allow a reduction of levodopa dosage and may reduce the dyskinesia and the fluctuations for a time. **Long-acting preparations** of Sinemet and Madopar (CR, controlled release) have promised a smoother effect; but in my experience they are often not satisfactory, since patients miss the anticipated surge of motor independence they have learned to expect for a short time after the dose of levodopa drugs. Doses of CR preparations have to be increased by about 30 to 50 per cent to secure the same effect as before, and often they fail to achieve it.

Afternoons are peculiarly troublesome, with patients often complaining that the lunchtime dose has failed to work. Disabling dyskinesia may paradoxically be prominent at such times—presumably an end-of-dose effect. It is said that dietary amino acids compete with levodopa drugs for absorption, thus reducing the effect perceived after lunch. **A low-protein meal** is occasionally successful in improving independence in the after-lunch period. If this is successful, the main meal of the day can be postponed to the evening dinner.

Drug holidays have been employed to try to rest or to re-set the dopaminergic receptors which have been overdriven by levodopa and other drugs, or to rid the brain of hypothetical toxic metabolites or false transmitters derived from these drugs: all unproven speculation. But in practice these only benefit sufferers who are plainly overdosed. This overdosage is evident in frequent and disabling dyskinesias and dystonias, often painful, during which parkinsonian signs are slight or inapparent.

Re-stabilization is then necessary, in hospital. We use hourly recording charts of the major parkinsonian signs, disability, mental performance, and side-effects. These observations usually reveal the problem, and then a modification of dosage or drug selection will sometimes be of benefit. The best initial strategy is to stop inessential or weakly-acting drugs and those medications given on equivocal indication for other ailments. The dose of levodopa is reduced by 50 to 75 per cent. Parkinsonian bradykinesia and rigidity emerge within a few days, but dyskinesia and dystonia generally disappear at the same time. The dose of levodopa is then cautiously increased by say 50 mg doses every three or four days until an acceptable degree of mobility is restored. This may be combined with a dopamine agonist, again introduced gradually. Simplification is the hallmark of effective therapeutics. At this stage the use of apomorphine may be of significant value to certain patients.

References

1. Ehringer, H. und Hornykiewicz, O. (1960). Verteilung von noradrenalin und dopamine (3-hydroxytryptamin) im gehirn des menschen und ihr verhalten bei erkrankungen des extra-pyramidalen systems. *Klinische Wochenschrift*, **38**, 1236–9.
2. Cotzias, G. C., Van Woert, M. H., and Schiffer, L. M. (1967). Aromatic amino acids and modification of Parkinsonism. *New England Journal of Medicine*, **276**, 374–9.
3. Yahr, M. D, Duvoisin, R. C., and Shear, M. J. (1969). Treatment of Parkinsonism with levodopa. *Archives of Neurology*, **21**, 343–54.
4. Rinne, U. K. (1978). Recent advances in research on Parkinsonism. *Acta Neurologica Scandinavica*, Suppl. .67, **57**, 77–113.

5. Barbeau, A. (1969). L-dopa therapy in Parkinson's disease. A critical review of nine years' experience. *Canadian Medical Association Journal*, **101**, 791–800.
6. Pearce, J. M. S. (1987). Modern treatment of Parkinson's disease. *British Journal of Hospital Medicine*, **37**, 59–66.
7. Cox, J. G. C., Pearce, I., Steiger, M., and Pearce, J. M. S. (1987). Disordered axial movement in Parkinson's disease. In *Parkinson's disease. Clinical and experimental advances*. (ed. F. C. Rose), pp. 71–5. John Libbey, London.
8. Melamed, E., Hefti, F., and Wurtman, R. J. (1980). Monoaminergic striatal neurons convert exogeneous L-dopa to dopamine in parkinsonism. *Annals of Neurology*, **8**, 558–63.
9. Marsden, C. D., Parkes, J. D., and Quinn, N. (1981). Fluctuations of disability in Parkinson's disease—clinical aspects. In *Movement disorders*, (ed. C. D. Marsden and S. Fahn), pp. 96–122. Butterworth Scientific, London.
10. Frankel, J. P., Pirtosek, Z., Bovington, R., Webster, R., Lees, A. J., and Stern, G. M. (1990). Diurnal differences in response to oral levodopa. *Journal of Neurology, Neurosurgery, and Psychiatry*, **53**, 948–50.
11. Shaw, K. M., Lees, A. J., and Stern, G. M. (1980). The impact of treatment with Levodopa on Parkinson's disease. *Quarterly Journal of Medicine*, New Series 59, No. **195**, 283–93.
12. Kempster, P. A., Frankel, J. P., Stern, G. M. and Lees, A. J. (1990). Comparison of motor response to apomorphine and levodopa in Parkinson's disease. *Journal of Neurology, Neurosurgery, and Psychiatry*, **53**, 1004–7.
13. Diamond, S., Markham, C., and Treciokas, L. J. (1978). A double-blind comparison of levodopa, Madopar, and Sinemet in Parkinson Disease. *Annals of Neurology*, **3**, 267–72.
14. Kempster, P. A., Frankel, J. P., Bovington, M., *et al.* (1989). Levodopa peripheral pharmacokinetics and duration of motor response in Parkinson's disease. *Journal of Neurology, Neurosurgery, and Psychiatry*, **52**, 718–23.
15. Marsden, C. D., and Parkes, J. D. (1976). 'On/Off' effects in patients with Parkinson's disease on chronic levodopa therapy. *Lancet*, **i**, 292–6.
16. Sage, J. I., Trooskin, S., Sonsalla, P. K., *et al.* (1988). Long term duodenal infusion of levodopa for motor fluctuations in parkinsonism. *Annals of Neurology* **24**, 87–9.
17. Marion, M. H., Stocchi, F., Quinn, N. P. *et al.* (1986). Repeated levodopa infusions in fluctuating Parkinson's disease: clinical and pharmacokinetic data. *Clinical Neuropharmacology*, **9**, 165–81.

12 Dopamine agonists: bromocriptine

The waning therapeutic effect attendant on long-term levodopa treatment encouraged a search for other drugs which could stimulate the dopaminergic drive in the striatum. Another incentive was provided by the troublesome dyskinesia, 'on–off' effects, and psychiatric sequelae of the levodopa drugs. It is when these symptoms of diminishing therapeutic benefit and intolerable fluctuations develop that it may be useful to add a dopamine agonist which stimulates or excites the dopamine receptors into greater activity.

The potential advantages are:

(1) that this group of agents do not require enzymes such as decarboxy-lases to convert precursors such as levodopa to active monoamines;

(2) that they do not compete with other amino acids for absorption at membrane barriers;

(3) that they are designed to act directly on specific dopamine receptors; and

(4) that by lowering rates of dopamine turnover, in theory they may produce less hydrogen peroxide and free radicals, and thus protect dopaminergic cells.

Dopamine receptors

Some of the characteristics of dopamine receptor function have been reviewed in Chapters 3 and 6, and the effects of levodopa therapy have been described in Chapter 11. Several dopamine receptors in the striatum have been characterized. D_1 receptors are linked to adenylate cyclase, and localized mainly on striatal neurons. D_2 receptors are not linked to adenylate cyclase, and are found mainly on descending cortical projections to the striatum. Presynaptic receptors also are demonstrable on nigrostriatal axons which have a negative or inhibitory feedback to the nigrostriatal neurons—impeding dopaminergic output.

In progressing disease the 80 per cent reduction in the number of dopaminergic neurons is accompanied by denervated postsynaptic receptors. Hypersensitivity of these receptors has been shown in experimental models, and has been considered to be the basis for drug-induced dyskinesia, and in neuroleptic-induced disease for akathisia and tardive dyskinesia.

In rats and primates with unilateral 6-OH-dopamine lesions causing parkinsonism the administration of dopamine agonists induces circling away from the denervated side in rats, whilst monkeys lose their tremor and may develop dyskinesia.[1,2] These effects can be inhibited by dopamine receptor blockade. Drugs that bind to receptors can be examined by radio-labelled dopamine receptor ligands; for example, H_3 dopamine an agonist, and H_3 haloperidol or H_3 spiropiperone—antagonists. Most available dopamine agonists are ergolenes, related to ergot derived from the fungus of the claviceps rye.

Bromocriptine pharmacology

Bromocriptine is a lysergic acid amide. It is currently the most popular dopamine agonist drug; lysuride and pergolide are the only alternatives currently available on prescription in the UK (Table 12.1). Like other agonists they are only effective in the presence of functional post-synaptic receptors. Bromocriptine acts by the stimulation of D_2 receptors. It is a mild D_1 antagonist. But it is also a mixed agonist–antagonist, with antagonist actions on brain-stem noradrenergic and serotoninergic receptors.

Absorption in man begins after about 20 to 40 minutes, with peak blood levels at 1 to 2 hours. Over 90 per cent undergoes first-pass

Table 12.1 Dopamine agonists (and a comparison with Madopar and Sinemet)

Drug	preparation	dose/pill	price/100*
Bromocriptine	tabs	1 mg	£9.28
Bromocriptine	tabs	2.5 mg	£18.07
Bromocriptine	caps	5 mg	£35.22
Bromocriptine	caps	10 mg	£65.16
Lysuride	tabs	200 μg	£24.00‡
Pergolide	tabs	1 mg	£150‡
Apomorphine	SC/inj	5 ml ampoule	£1244†
Madopar	caps	200/50	£22.46
Sinemet	tabs	250/25	£17.87

*Actual cost varies with dose and frequency. Prices cited are for UK (MIMS, Oct. 1991).
†Hospital price per 100 ampoules.
‡Lysuride daily dosage up to 1 to 5 mg; pergolide 2 to 5 mg.

hepatic metabolism. Its plasma half-life is around 7 hours, which is twice that of Sinemet. The duration of clinical improvement is variable, but of the order of 6 to 8 hours. It has been utilized clinically as early monotherapy, late monotherapy, and (most commonly) in conjunction with levodopa drugs.

Combined therapy: bromocriptine with levodopa drugs

When it was introduced in the mid-1970s treatment was most commonly started in levodopa failures.[3,4] At this stage the nigrostriatal pathway has been bombarded with levodopa-derived dopamine for several years. The effects of such secondary or late use of bromocriptine should be separated from its early use as monotherapy in 'levodopa virgins'. In secondary cases, it is added to the existing dose of Sinemet or Madopar. It is started in small doses of 2.5 mg daily, and slowly increased every week or so until benefit is apparent. This usually means a total dose of 20 to 60 mg/day—if side-effects permit. As benefit starts, it may be possible to reduce the levodopa dose by about 10–25 per cent. This addition often affords a useful improvement in antiparkinsonian efficacy, and the small reduction of levodopa is useful in reducing dyskinesia, dystonias, and fluctuations. Bromocriptine is a potent drug which may reduce all the symptoms of Parkinson's disease; but its side-effects can be prohibitive.

Lieberman and colleagues[5] summarize studies involving 790 patients. Improvement was judged to have occurred in 489 (61 per cent), adverse effects in 217 (27 per cent). In low dosage (below 20 mg/day) the drug has weak effects; in doses of 30 to 100 mg/day it has definite anti-parkinsonian activity approximating in potency to the levodopa preparations. But toxicity is a serious problem in over 25 per cent of patients.

In low-dose studies (average 16 mg/day) without levodopa improvement was claimed in 58 per cent of 79 patients; only 9 per cent had adverse effects—but most of the subjects studied had mild or early disease. In an open study we were unable to demonstrate adequate clinical efficacy in doses of less than 20 mg/day.

In seven studies of high-dose treatments (average 48 mg/day) combined with levodopa, improvement was noted in 58 per cent of 367 patients, with adverse effects in 32 per cent; most subjects had advanced disease. Trials comparing bromocriptine alone with high-dose bromocriptine plus levodopa show very similar improvement rates, confirming the potency of the drug (Table 12.2).

One of the advantages discovered in practice is that bromocriptine alone in the patient who has not received levodopa does not produce

Table 12.2 Comparison of clinical condition between patients treated with bromocriptine plus levodopa drugs (Lieberman *et al.* 1990)[5] [composite results]

Drug	patients no.	duration PD (years)	mild/mod (% of patients)	improved (% of patients)	toxic (% of patients)
BC alone	222	4.8	72	60	21
BC/LD	568	10	21	63	30
BC low/LD	280	7.5	45	68	21
BC high/LD	510	9.1	36	59	31

BC = bromocriptine; LD = levodopa drugs.

early, serious fluctuations or 'on–off' swings. Further, dyskinesia is much less frequent and severe in patients on bromocriptine alone. These benefits have to be balanced by the higher incidence of what in my experience are also more severe psychiatric sequelae.

Early monotherapy

Rinne[6] has advocated the early use of bromocriptine alone, when others would have started to introduce Madopar or Sinemet. If the total benefit of the latter is related to the duration of treatment (that is, a given patient has a fixed period of say six years' useful response to Madopar), then the initial use of bromocriptine alone will in theory extend the total useful period of therapeutic benefit. Long-term use of low-dose bromocriptine given in early cases produces few dyskinetic or 'on–off' side-effects, but the treatment has been disappointing in that most patients require a levodopa drug as an adjunct. An alternative strategem is to use both drugs from the start, but to employ lower than normal doses of each: an attempt to buy the best of both worlds with minimal toxicity. The UK Bromocriptine Research Group treated 134 patients in a double-blind study, comparing a low/slow regime, building up to a maximum of 25 mg/day, with a high/fast group, increasing up to 100 mg/day, over 26 weeks.[7] The regime was a failure in 4 per cent of the high/fast group and in 13 per cent of the low/slow group; toxicity necessitated withdrawal of treatment in 19 of the high/fast group and in 15 of the low/slow group. In an open pilot study in levodopa virgins, we found no clinically significant responses in doses of less than 20 mg/day treated for periods of up to 28 months.[8] Patients treated with doses of 25 to 40 mg/day showed useful improvements in Webster scores and in overall motor performance in 40 per cent of the subjects, which were sustained for 12 to 27 months. Intolerable psychosis or inadequate control of motor symptoms necessitated withdrawal in 40 per cent of patients. Slow introduction with 1.25 mg/day increasing by 1.25 mg/week was better tolerated than the more rapid introduction and increase by 2.5 mg/week. These low-dose treatment devices are of dubious value so far, and before they can be recommended the results of other trials must be awaited.

Adverse effects of bromocriptine

The most common side-effects are nausea, vomiting, dyspepsia, hypotension, hallucinations, psychosis, and dyskinesias. In long-term use we see cramps and pains in the legs, often at night, with or without obvious claudication. A curiously hard brawny oedema is occasionally encountered. Adverse effects improve on withdrawing the drug, but psychosis in my experience can be serious in degree and take a long time to subside. Dyspepsia and gastro-oesophageal reflux trouble a minority of patients; the occasional resurgence of pre-treatment peptic ulcer symptoms is encountered. The possibility of vasospastic coronary or peripheral vascular complications should be remembered with any ergot-type drug.

Bromocriptine causes more severe psychiatric complications than levodopa drugs. These are most commonly nightmares, wanderings, confusion, and delusions, and amount to frank psychosis in a number of patients; aggressive psychosis can be difficult to manage and may persist for many days even after the dosage has been reduced to below what has previously been well tolerated. These complications may be reversible on reducing the dose; but often it is necessary to stop the drug. They are especially likely in the over-seventies and in those with previous confusion or dementia, but can occur in younger subjects in their fifties and sixties. Used alone, bromocriptine is satisfactory in only about one-third of patients.

In general, bromocriptine should not be given to the geriatric age-group, and treatment should preferably be supervised by a neurological specialist. It can be recommended in late levodopa failures. We employ bromocriptine in moderate dosage (for example, building up slowly to 20 to 40 mg/day in an attempt to minimize toxicity), aiming at improved physical independence and reduction in dyskinesias by continuing Madopar/Sinemet in doses reduced by 10 to 25 per cent.

Other dopamine agonists

Several other ergolene drugs have been examined. Their modes of action as postsynaptic dopamine agonists (receptor agonists of D_1, D_2, or both) are the same as those of bromocriptine, their potencies are of the same order, and they produce similar toxicity, with the exception of lergotrile, which is hepatotoxic. Lysuride and pergolide are mentioned specifically, since they are now available in the UK, but the other drugs are not currently licensed or marketed for general use. They are listed below:

Lergotrile (D_2 agonist), dose 50 mg/day is markedly hepatotoxic.

Mesulergine (D_1 and D_2 agonist), dose 7–27 mg/day, provokes testicular tumours in rats, but not in man; clinical studies have ceased.

Lysuride

Lysuride is an ergoline compound which excites postsynaptic striatal dopamine D_2 receptors. It also has high affinity for 5-HT receptors. It is well absorbed by the oral route. It produces variable peak plasma concentrations. Several trials have attested to its potential efficacy. Its application is currently in late levodopa failures, where it shows antiparkinsonian activity of the same potency as bromocriptine or pergolide. Lieberman and colleagues[5] summarized 7 studies including 315 patients. The mean dose of lysuride was 2.2 mg (range 1.2–4.7 mg), and improvement was claimed in 221/315 (70 per cent) of patients, with a range of 57 to 92 per cent. In most cases lysuride was added to levodopa. Toxicity is appreciable, some 23 per cent of patients needing to stop medication because of mental changes, dyskinesias, and postural hypotension. Overall clinical efficacy seems to be equivalent to that of bromocriptine.

Pergolide

Pergolide is a synthetic ergoline, a potent direct dopamine agonist (D_1, D_2, and D_3 receptors),[9] which unlike bromocriptine does not require the release of presynaptic dopamine. Rapidly absorbed, it produces peak plasma concentrations at 60 to 120 minutes. Its half-life is about 27 hours, but its antiparkinsonian action is from 5 to 9 hours. It is gradually introduced—using 50 μg *nocte* for 3 nights, then increases of 100 to 150 μg every third day, and then 250μg increases every third day to a maintenance dose of 2 to 5 mg/day in three divided doses. It may allow reduction of concomitant levodopa drugs by one-third to one-half, with improvement in disability and in the 'off' time. Benefit may wane in some patients after a year. As monotherapy it has yielded disappointing results, but more experience is needed.

Side-effects are similar to those of bromocriptine—nausea,

hallucinosis, dyskinesia, sedation, and postural hypotension. Its longer duration of action is its main attraction.

Apomorphine

Apomophine is an old drug first used by Schwab in 1951. It is a potent direct-acting D_1 and D_2 striatal receptor agonist. It does not depend on the same central or peripheral pharmacokinetic mechanisms as levodopa. The efficacy of apomorphine depends on the integrity of the postsynaptic receptors in the striatum. Its ability to produce clinically optimal activity at this site is probably equivalent to that of a single dose of levodopa/DDI, provided that adequate absorption and transport of the latter are maximal at the critical time. It is useful in patients with declining motor responses, and in those with intractable 'on–off' fluctuations,[10] and does not appear to decrease in efficacy or dopaminergic action with repeated dosage.

It is given subcutaneously by a pump, or more often by injections, which some patients or relatives can be taught to administer. These are placed in the abdominal wall, thighs, or buttocks. Intranasal administration with a metered dose of solution containing 10 mg/ml has been shown to be feasible in small numbers of subjects,[11] and certainly mucosal absorption has been demonstrated. More extensive trials are needed; but, if confirmed, this route could be a convenient improvement over subcutaneous injections.

Apomorphine causes vomiting unless each dose is preceded by Domperidone (20 mg tds, orally), a potent antiemetic drug. The injections usually produce obvious benefit in 5–10 minutes; this lasts for 40 to 80 minutes—a short period, but one which affords the patient a more predictable lease of independent activity three or four times each day, and at times of his or her choice. Effective dosage varies from 2 mg up to 10 mg, and has to be determined by trial and error. Frequency varies with patients' demands, but is commonly three times per day, given during the 'off' state; and some patients seem happy to self-inject up to six times each day. Allergic reactions are rare, but local pain and erythema at the site of injection is occasionally a nuisance—one which should lead to frequent changes in the site of injection.

Experimentally, it can be shown that oscillations can be overcome by continuous stimulation of the dopamine receptors. This has been achieved by intravenous levodopa infusions for several days and by intraduodenal infusions. Neither method is practical or acceptable to many patients; but further assessment of the duodenal route may yield advantages for patients otherwise disabled or chairbound. Apomorphine represents a practical alternative.

References

1. Fuxe, K., Agnati, L. F., and Kohler, C. (1981). Characterisation of normal and supersensitive dopamine receptors: effects of ergot drugs and neuropeptides. *Journal of Neural Transmitters*, **51**, 3–37.
2. Goldstein, M., Lew, J. Y., Sauter, A., and Lieberman, A. (1980). The affinities of ergot compounds for dopamine agonist and antagonist receptor sites. In *Ergot compounds and brain functions: neuroendocrine and neuropsychiatric aspects* (ed. M. Goldstein), pp. 75–82. Raven Press, New York.
3. Calne, D. B., Teychenne, P. F., Claveira, L. E., *et al.* (1974). Bromocriptine in parkinsonism. *British Medical Journal*, **2**, 442–4.
4. Pearce, I. and Pearce, J. M. S. (1978). Bromocriptine in Parkinsonism. *British Medical Journal*, **1**, 1402–4.
5. Lieberman, A. N., Gopinathan, G., Neophytides, A., Nelson, J., and Goldstein, M. (1990). Dopamine agonists in Parkinson's disease. In *Parkinson's disease.* (ed. G. M. Stern), pp. 509–37. Chapman and Hall Medical, London.
6. Rinne, U. K. (1986). Dopamine agonists as primary treatment in Parkinson's disease. *Advances in Neurology*, **45**, 519–23.
7. UK Bromocriptine Research Group (1989). Bromocriptine in Parkinson's disease: a double-blind study comparing 'low–slow' and 'high–fast' introductory dosage regimens in *de novo* patients. *Journal of Neurology, Neurosurgery, and Psychiatry*, **52**, 77–82.
8. Pearce, I. and Pearce, J. M. S. (1985). Low-dose bromocriptine in Parkinson's disease. *Journal of Neurology, Neurosurgery, and Psychiatry*, **48**, 388–9.
9. Langtry, H. D. and Clissold, S. P. (1990). Pergolide: a review of its pharmacological properties and therapeutic potential in Parkinson's disease. *Drugs*, **39**, 491–506.
10. Gancher, S. T., Woodward, W. R., Boucher, B., and Nutt, J. G. (1989). Peripheral pharmacokinetics of apomorphine in humans. *Annals of Neurology*, **26**, 232–8.
11. Kapoor, R., Turjanski, N., Frankel, J. *et al.* (1990). Intranasal apomorphine: a new treatment in Parkinson's disease. *Journal of Neurology, Neurosurgery, and Psychiatry*, **53**, 1015.

13 Surgery for Parkinson's disease

Stereotactic surgery

Surgical treatment for Parkinson's disease is now rarely recommended. Thirty years ago there was a vogue for placing tiny destructive lesions in the basal ganglia by means of a 'stereotactic apparatus' which permitted very accurate placement of the lesion in the pallidum and later in the ventrolateral nucleus of the thalamus. Chemicals (alcohol, chemopallidectomy), and hot (thermocoagulation) and cold (cryocoagulation) probes were later used. These methods were fairly effective in controlling refractory unilateral tremor and rigidity. Stereotactic surgery was of no benefit to the facial expression, weak voice, slowness of movement, stooped posture, and tendency to fall—the so-called central features of the disease. Indeed, sometimes these symptoms were made worse—in at least 15 per cent of patients.[1] The initial improvement was not always maintained. Buren and colleagues found that three years after thalamotomy the disease had progressed and the disability exceeded the initial functional benefit.[2] Some patients showed mental decline, not evident in the preoperative assessment.

Surgery is still used, especially in Japan, for early one-sided tremor and rigidity, if patients fail to respond to other measures. Narabayashi claims that the introduction of microelectrodes, targeting, and the production of more accurate and discrete (4–5 mm) lesions has allowed a 'much higher percentage of superior results' and fewer complications. Lesions in the Vim thalamic nucleus are selected for tremor, and lesions in the Vo-complex for rigidity. Narabayashi[3] stresses the different types of akinesia and their relevance to surgical outcome. Slowness of movement and impaired co-ordination he associates with rigidity, and finds that they are relieved by surgery. Poverty of movement not due to coincident rigidity is unaffected. Freezing of gait and festination are unaffected. Stereotactic thalamotomy, was fashionable between 1957 and 1972, but in most specialized centres in the UK and USA it is now seldom used, since levodopa drugs, despite their shortcomings, in general have proved effective.

Nigral transplants

In 1981 in Sweden the first attempts were made to transplant the patient's own adrenal medulla (autografts) into the caudate nucleus, a part of the basal ganglia which is involved in the transmission of dopamine. The adrenal medulla is rich in amines, including dopamine. The hope was that this would bypass immunological rejection and provide an added source of natural dopamine. Results in patients were disappointingly slight, and any doubtful benefit wore off quickly.[4] This work showed, however, that the surgery was feasible. Later, transplants of fetal dopamine neurons in the caudate head and in the putamen have been performed, and Lindvall and others have shown that the tissue took on its new blood supply and to some extent formed new tyrosine-hydroxylase functioning nerve connections in the receptor site.[5]

More publicity was given to the extension of this work in Mexico in younger patients with Parkinson's disease. Two of the twelve patients treated died within six months, but from unrelated causes. Benefit was claimed for rigidity, akinesia, and tremor; but improvement was variable, and was delayed from three to ten months, and in some cases for more than a year. There was no controlled series, and the florid publicity in the national press caused more than a little sceptical criticism amongst neuroscientists in the USA. Isolated reports of similar procedures in North America have confirmed the soundness of this cautious reception. Subsequent operations transplanting the adrenal have shown variable and slight benefits, with increasing periods of activity and less akinetic 'off' periods in each 24 hours. In many cases, it affords no reduction of antiparkinsonian drugs, and the morbidity after operation can be considerable.[3] For the moment, except in Mexico, this approach has been abandoned. Other surgical methods have been attempted, notably the transplantation of fetal substantia nigra. This area is the main focus of loss of dopamine stores in human Parkinson's disease, so it makes good sense to replace it with the same tissue.

The number of operations performed has been very small, largely because it involves major surgery, and because there are ethical problems in using fetal donor tissue. The results are not yet proven. Strict scientific control comparing operated against non-operated cases of similar age, sex, and severity of illness is essential before we can say that the operation is useful in certain types or stages of the disease, or that it is of no benefit to any patient. Madrazo's most recent report (October 1990) claims that:[6]

'the fact that roughly 25–30% of those who have received transplants benefit from them justifies further experimental clinical transplantations. Of the 41 patients to whom we have given autotransplants or fetal homotransplants, 30% have not responded and 10% have been 'harmed', after a follow up of two or more years; 60% have shown appreciable signs of functional recovery and improved quality of life over two to four years. In addition, in those patients who did not respond the rate of progression of the disease may [sic] have been slowed.'

Many workers in this field would have reservations about the accuracy and objectivity of these results at this juncture. At the moment these techniques are exciting, but must be viewed with cautious optimism.

It is not known whether transplantation alters the evolution or outcome of Parkinson's disease, it is not known whether any such benefit will be lasting. And it is not known whether the unknown agent(s) which primarily initiate the disease will also destroy the graft. We must also remember that Parkinson's disease reflects a disorder not only of dopamine, but of many other neurotransmitter systems, which may not be replaced by the grafts, even if they function. These techniques hold out promise, and should not be dismissed because of the present lack of evidence of unequivocal efficacy. They must be scientifically tested. Meanwhile, no patient should feel deprived of an implant until we have far more information.

References

1. Cooper, I. S., Riklan, M., Stellar, *et al.* (1968). A multidisciplinary investigation of neurosurgical rehabilitation in bilateral parkinsonism. *Journal of the American Geriatric Society*, **16**, 1177–306.
2. Van Buren, J. Li, C. L., Shapiro, D. *et al.* (1973). A qualitative and quantitative evaluation of parkinsonians three to six years following thalamotomy. *Confin Neurology*, **35**, 202–35.
3. Narabayashi, H. (1989). Stereotaxic Vim thalamotomy for treatment of tremor. *European Neurology*, **29**, Suppl. 29–31.
4. Goetz, C. G. *et al.* (1989). Multicenter study of autologous adrenal medullary transplantation to the corpus striatum in patients with advanced Parkinson's disease. *New England Journal of Medicine*, **320**, 337–42.
5. Lindvall, O., Brundin, P., Widner, H., *et al.* (1990). Grafts of fetal dopamine neurons survive and improve motor function in Parkinson's disease. *Science*, **247**, 574–7.
6. Madrazo, I., Aguilera, M., and Franco-Bourland, R. (1990). Cell implantation in Parkinson's disease. (Letter). *British Medical Journal* **301**, 874.

14 Other treatments, social problems, and terminal care

Although drug treatment is the most important single measure in reversing the symptoms and disabilities of Parkinson's disease, there is far more to the treatment of the patient than the administration of drugs alone. The author claims no expertise in the individual techniques employed by ancillary therapists, and seeks only to point to the principal measure available which are used in conjunction with medical treatments.

This chapter is written with patients and their families in mind as possible readers.

Many of the problems faced by sufferers are not due to Parkinson's disease itself, but to the coincidental accompanying conditions from which many people suffer; these may need separate medical attention. Some patients are diabetic, some have high blood pressure, some asthma, some heart disease or bronchitis; and many have arthritis. Thus the care of the whole individual is essential.

Identifying the problems

Certain problems commonly occur in Parkinson's disease; the first step is to identify them, and the second to try to find the means of helping to correct them.

The following are some common parkinsonian problems which patients may identify:

Walking slowly, with short, shuffling steps; finding oneself stopping or hesitating when walking through doorways; finding one's feet freezing to the floor, and one's writing getting smaller, and shaky and spidery; and difficulties experienced in turning in a narrow space without falling; getting out of a chair; swinging the arms naturally and unselfconsciously when walking; standing up straight rather than hunched forwards; turning over in bed; getting on and off a toilet; using the hands for fine manipulations, as in writing, using a screwdriver, sewing on buttons, or crocheting; and getting one's arms in or out of a dress, shirt, or jacket.

Physiotherapy

Physiotherapy has specific benefits for particular problems; it also has a generally beneficial effect in boosting morale—in persuading the patient that something active is being done, and that he/she is playing an active part in the treatment. The general benefit is much influenced by the personality and the attitude of both patient and therapist.

Bad habits are better eradicated early than late. As a result of advanced illness, however, motivation may be poor and memory and concentration impaired, and effective co-operation may be impossible.

Assessment is the first step. This includes: the physical disabilities, learning capacity and mental state, home circumstances, and availability of able-bodied friends and family to continue to carry out any instructions.

Occupational therapy. A home visit with an occupational therapist is invaluable, and he/she will usually prepare a report for the hospital consultant describing specific problems, the need for gadgets, hand rails, high seats, and other provisions. A wide range of home aids is available: some to be purchased privately, many available on the National Health Scheme.

Exercises. Aims are to: correct abnormal gait, correct bad posture, prevent or minimize stiffness and contractures of the joints, improve use and facilities of the limbs, and provide a regime which can be used at home by the patient. Regular exercise is beneficial whenever disabilities permit. It helps to maintain muscle tone and strength and to prevent contractures and stiffening. Walking is one of the most useful exercises. Most people in the early stages of Parkinsons' disease can walk a mile or two each day—sometimes much more. A conscious effort should be made to keep the back straight, with shoulders back and head upright, and to take long, slow strides. Even patients more severely affected by the disease can often walk three or four hundred yards, and perhaps repeat this once or twice every day. Slippy surfaces, snow, ice, and wet leaves should obviously be avoided.

The physiotherapist will concentrate on teaching the patient to sit straight, often in a high upright chair, aided by a cushion in the back. She or he will show how to concentrate on striking the heel down when walking, and how to improve moving from sitting to standing by pulling the heels in under the front edge of the chair and throwing the weight forwards as the patient gets up.

Standing in front of a long mirror may help the patient to see and correct any stoop or bent posture of the neck and trunk. Individual exercises are aimed to help balance, lengthen the patient's stride, and perhaps relieve the pain of a frozen shoulder—a common complication. Constant repetition and practice are necessary at home, especially when the therapist is no longer badgering the patient. There is no substitute for the 'do it yourself' attitude! Exercises may be made easier and more rhythmical if performed to music on a cassette or radio. Visits to out-patient therapy may be helpful, and encouragement may be obtained by group exercises.

'Therapeutic holidays' organized by the Parkinson's Disease Society combine physiotherapy, occupational therapy, and speech therapy on an intensive basis. As the disease progresses some require aids to facilitate activity.

Physical aids and appliances

Walking-sticks add to stability and are socially unobtrusive, but should not be advocated too early, because patients may see them as a sign of impending deterioration and failure. A tripod held in one hand does the same thing on a wider base. Zimmer frames are not recommended, except as a short-term measure when mobilizing after injury or operation in hospital: they break the natural rhythm of walking. If, however, they are fitted with wheels and hand-brakes, they can be valuable. Delta frames with two 'legs' and a front wheel, or a rolator with two legs and two wheels, can also be very helpful. Brakes add to the sense of security.

Manual dexterity may be improved by practice with blocks, jigsaws, and certain games. Grab-rails fitted near the patient's bed and in the lavatory and bathroom are often necessary to prevent falls and injury. Buttons and zips can be replaced by velcro fasteners. Casual or elastic-sided shoes or trainers may be much easier than lace-up shoes. Large-handled knives, forks, and spoons and stick-on plates and egg-cups can save spills. Many of these can be supplied or recommended by the occupational therapist. The Welfare Department of the Parkinson's Disease Society is also able to advise.

Speech therapy

Many victims of the disease are embarrassed and frustrated by their speech. It may be slurred and hesitant, with lack of variation in pitch and volume of the voice. Assessment by a speech therapist will examine the way the patient breathes and moves the lips, tongue, and jaw in the formation of speech: all elements which we perform unconsciously or automatically.

Speech therapists identify defects in respiratory pattern, often with poor expiratory function. There is difficulty in synchronizing the expiratory passage of air with phonation. Poor control of the air stream makes the initiation of speech difficult, and the volume of voice-production sounds weak and strained; impaired control of the air passage embarrasses the modulation of volume and the loudness of phonation; and leads to a monotonous voice quality. Articulation by the lips, tongue, and jaw is impaired by the defects in the motor control of the muscles of the face, jaw, and larynx. Articulation of single sounds and short words may be preserved, but the combinations and sequences of sound production in longer phrases or sentences are often impaired by the striatal defect of control of the muscles involved. Intelligibility is marred by speech which is too slow or too fast, or by an articulation which gains in speed—as in festination of gait. Reduced emphasis and inadequate stress placed in pausing between words or phrases (prosody) hampers understanding. Word stress may be completely lost. Contrasting tone and stress destroy normal emphasis and intelligibility; even syllables within a word may lack the essential emphasis and may be inappropriate. Variation in pitch is also lacking, and contributes the monotonous lack of varied intonation.

In summary, the control of the voice is deficient and produces a monotonous pitch, lack of timbre and volume control, and lack of stress on certain sounds. The voice sounds hoarse and quiet.

Speech therapy may utilize delayed audio-feedback (DAF), in which the patients hear their own speech after a measured latent interval; this can be used to modify and improve voice and speech output. Scott and Caird[1] introduced prosodic exercises to patients treated at home for two to three weeks. Intonation, stress, and rhythm were practised, and patients were encouraged to recognize the abnormal prosody of their speech. Therapy included a voice-operated visual reinforcement device, the 'Vocalite'; but this proved to be of limited value. Other therapists have concentrated on improving the capacity and control of breathing and co-ordination and control of voice-production, emphasizing pitch variation and loudness, intonation, and stress patterns. Delayed auditory feedback may help individuals with marked slurring, dysarthria and palilalia, improving prosody, loudness, and pitch. This and other manoeuvres to a modest extent can help to retrain the voice and speech; but dramatic improvements are not common.

Communication aids include 'Edu–Com scanning', a device to point to a word or picture, showing the patient's intention and meaning. The 'Microwriter' links a TV and a printer or speech synthesizer, and can be of occasional help to patients when speech training is unsuccessful.

It is of enormous advantage if there is good liaison between the hospital-based physiotherapist, the occupational therapist, the social worker, and the ward team. They will meet to discuss plans and joint assessments when patients are admitted to the ward, and will continue supervision, where possible, after the patient goes home. They will also link up with the GP and district welfare services. A useful information pack for patients and therapists is available from the Parkinson's Disease Society.

Driving

Slowness in initiating movement is an obvious danger to the Parkinsonian patient who is driving any type of motorized vehicle, as well as to other road users. Slow reaction times may hamper the rapid application of brakes or steering necessary to avoid disaster in an emergency. Tremor alone seldom interferes with movements, and is not in itself a contraindication to driving. Wild fluctuations in performance as in 'on–off' swings may suddenly impair a driver's control over his or her vehicle. Dyskinesia and dystonia may interfere with control of foot pedals. Despite these obvious hazards, notifications by the police to the Department of Transport about parkinsonian patients are rare.[2] Early disease is notifiable to the DVLA as a 'prospective disability', which should not ban the patient, but should necessitate regular neurological review, with limitation of the licence to three years, subject to medical assessment.

Evaluation of fitness to drive is not easy, and is always to some extent a subjective decision. There is considerable variation from hour to hour, even from minute to minute. Laboratory studies of motor skills, reaction times, and vigilance give little direct information about the actuality of driving performance and reactions. Microcomputers producing simulated driving conditions and measuring responses such as steering, braking and acceleration have been performed,[3] yet there remains doubt as to how well these tests correlate with the potential for driving errors. Experts have concluded that there is no substitute for individual consultation and advice on adaptations; the Department of Transport provides mobility advice and vehicle information, but this does not constitute an assessment of safety.

In practice many patients have sufficient insight and sense to relinquish driving when properly cautioned. Spouses are often good witnesses as to safety and speed of reaction in a crisis, and will report erratic or worrying performance. The physician should use his or her authority to prohibit driving under these circumstances and advise patients to notify the DVLA. On occasions, when in doubt, a short journey by the doctor in the passenger seat may tell all.

There is some evidence that parkinsonians are cautious, and may even have fewer accidents than others,[1] possibly by limiting their speed and distances, and by avoiding motorways and night driving. When there is marked bradykinesia, poor speed and co-ordination of hand and foot tapping, rapid 'on–off' swings, or any appreciable cognitive defect, patients should be plainly advised against driving; most early cases, however, are fit to drive, often for several years.

Practical problems

Driving may be facilitated by automatic transmission, which is especially helpful if tremor or bradykinesia predominate in the left leg. Bradykinesia of the arms and hands is not countered by manual controls, which are not a practical solution.

Those whose work or leisure is dependent on writing or draughtsmanship may find assistance from a sloping desk top, and through the use of squared or lined paper. Desk-top computers and word processors are within the capabilities of many patients; the ability to correct material on the screen before printing it increases efficiency, and may save unwanted frustration and expletives. Patients repeatedly report the advantages they have found from reporting their illness to family and friends, and selectively to employers, rather than concealing it. A patient recently remarked that 'flexible attitudes, understanding, and consideration do help!' At a stage when the pressures and demands of work prove too great a number of patients set up as freelance agents in their own area of skill, and succeed in circumstances where they can determine their own patterns of work, travelling, and rest, freed of the pressures from employers and from colleagues in the same job. Many seek early retirement; but this decision must be founded on the many factors peculiar to the individual. In general, work, mental occupation, and mixing with others are beneficial in maintaining physical activity, motivation, and a regular timetable; but there comes a time for some patients when the strains incurred are intolerable. Alternative lighter work and self-employment are feasible for some younger subjects; retirement is necessary in others, but should be carefully planned, with the emphasis on widening the scope of leisure activities rather than on retreating to a comfy armchair.

Some general observations

Activity is the keynote throughout the illness. 'Do as much as you can', is sensible counsel; three walks of 400 yards each are at least as beneficial as one of 1200 yards. Patients will also have to make certain adjustments to their life-styles; but these are usually obvious, and changes are gradual, so that they have plenty of time to make these alterations. Patients may have to allow a little longer for getting dressed or going to work, or for planning and packing for holidays or journeys. It may take two goes to mow the lawn, instead of one. A little planning in advance, allowing more time, will make most tasks possible.

Prohibitions of sexual activities are inappropriate, and many patients enjoy normal sexual practices until advancing disease or age reduces their libido or potency.

It is prudent to avoid fanatical or crackpot schemes that patients read about, and to eschew gossip from certain glossy magazines or well-meaning but ill-informed neighbouring do-gooders. A lot of money can be wasted on charlatan remedies, health foods, acupuncture, osteopathy, and so forth. Medical opinion should have no rooted objections to these therapies, but does not employ them unless they have been carefully and scientifically tested, so that it is clear if they are of benefit or not.

Patients with Parkinson's disease require no special diets, but should have a balanced, enjoyable diet, with fresh meat, fish, fruit, and vegetables, like everyone else. Alcoholic drinks are not prohibited. In certain instances the timing and content of meals may be altered by the physician to assist the absorption of levodopa drugs. With the help of the GP patients should obtain up-to-date medical support and supervision of their drug treatment, and advice about any possible side-effects.

More specialized guidance is available from consultant clinics, private and NHS, which will also supervise most patients where staffing levels and facilities permit. The spouse or partner's presence is of great advantage to the physician and the patient in many consultations. Modern sociologists pay much attention to 'caring for the carers'. The spouse may come to adopt a dominant role and may have problems in coming to terms with the illness and its ramifications into normal family life. Many adapt remarkably well, and some thrive on their new-found role. Others are less resilient, and will require much encouragement, guidance, and support from the medical team.

The welfare services and hospital units also provide support from physiotherapists, occupational therapists, and social workers when the need arises; but currently the provision and quality of support is variable.

Advancing disability and terminal care

The ravages of advancing disease will eventually deprive many patients of mobility and physical independence. Some manage in their own homes for many years, others without adequate family help are cared for in a variety of residential homes, nursing homes, and geriatric wards. Standards vary widely. Such patients may have severe disabilities, but many are not terminal. Psychological factors are pre-eminent, determining the quality of life at a time when physical hardships impose such grave strictures. Depression, confusional states, and dementia pose serious problems. At this stage drugs should be appraised; many will be found unnecessary and should be stopped. If, despite antiparkinsonian medication given in the optimal tolerated dosage, the patient is barely able to stand and is unable to walk; the drugs can often be discontinued without physical deterioration. Symptomatic treatment for other ailments should in like fashion be reviewed and minimized or stopped—provided this is compatible with the patient's comfort. Surprising improvement in alertness and appetite may ensue, and a sleepy apathetic state may sometimes disappear.

Terminal care

If I had strength enough to hold a pen I would write how easy and pleasant a thing it is to die.

William Hunter

At a later stage patients appear to be nearing the end of life. Although this is nowadays often occasioned by disorders other than their Parkinson's disease, the principles of terminal treatment[4] are the same in either case.

Adequate 'support systems' are sadly lacking in some circumstances, and idle words and platitudes may prove to be pie in the sky. The aim is to keep the patient comfortable, alert, and free of troublesome symptoms, both physical and mental. The ill and aged may have a low tolerance for minor 'nuisance symptoms' which compound their miseries; paradoxically, if they are demented, their awareness and thereby their suffering may be much less, but a source of distress and sometimes guilt for their relatives. In the treatment of the earlier stages of the illness, we may rightly seek for a personal trust and faith from the patient, based on the broad eclecticism of the dedicated physician, and to this end we may eschew the multi-disciplinary approach. However, in the later stages, when serious disability dominates the scene, the help of a team of therapists and carers may become imperative.

Personal worries, family considerations, and financial obligations may all serve to add to the sufferer's plight. Emotional support and attention to personal worries are necessary. Friends, family, and the patient's minister may all give invaluable help.

When possible, most patients are happier ending their days at home, with their family, surrounded by familiar faces and their own possessions. Every possible means should be sought to attain this end. Relatives, fearful of the responsibility and of their own ability to cope, may be aided and encouraged by a concerted effort to provide the necessary home nursing and social services. It is helpful to be able to offer respite in hospital for a time, in the event of breakdown of provisions and care at home. The family doctor plays a vital role in his knowledge of the quality of local facilities; he will often make the appropriate arrangements for attendance at day centres and the provision of carers, and give his own invaluable brand of expertise, relief, and encouragement.

Hospital treatment has benefited by the experience learned from the better hospices. Time spent with patients and with the family is a costly and precious commodity. Loneliness can be in some measure overcome by group activities of compatible patients, but little is gained by surrounding a television set with a group of uninterested patients, each carefully ignoring the box, preoccupied by his or her own sad plight. The family can be involved in the ward in some circumstances; this is often of benefit to the patient, fosters a constructive co-operation with nursing and other staff, and permits informal discussions of current and future problems.

Drugs

The ideal is to simplify, minimize, or abolish those drugs which are not demonstrably benefiting the patient's symptoms. Nonetheless, certain drugs are needed in some sufferers to ensure their well-being. In the preterminal phase it is usually an advantage to stop specific anti-parkinsonian drugs—anticholinergics and levodopa drugs. But there may be occasional circumstances where intractable dribbling is best controlled by tiny doses of benztropine or orphenadrine, or painful rigidity by tiny doses of levodopa drugs; each patient needs an individual consideration of his symptoms.

Drugs for other ailments, for example hypotensive drugs, may well be dispensed with. The advent of other symptoms may require small doses of drugs to afford control and contentment. Pain is not a major feature of terminal Parkinson's disease, but coincident arthritis or metastatic disease may demand analgesics, which should never be spared at this stage. Frequent small doses to prevent pain are preferable to the relief of established pain. Aspirin, paracetamol, codeine, and if necessary morphine solution 5–10 mg, given 4-hourly will often be effective. MST continus 10–20 mg, given 12-hourly is a useful alternative. Suppositories of oxycodone can be useful if oral preparations are not tolerated. Larger doses of morphine or heroin should never be withheld if pain is incompletely suppressed.

Nausea and vomiting may complicate many other illnesses in their terminal phases. Antiemetics are valuable, and any dopamine-blocking action (for example, with phenothiazines) should be ignored unless there is significant worsening of the patient's complaints. Domperidone 10–20 mg tds, or metoclopramide 10 mg tds are suitable. The aim is to keep symptoms at bay by the minimum pharmacotherapy necessary to do so. Polypharmacy is as ill-advised in terminal care as it is in other circumstances.

Common coincidental symptoms arising in the elderly include nausea and vomiting, which can be relieved by adjustments of diet, by antacids, or by metoclopramide. Abdominal pain, hiccup, anorexia, and constipation will require attention to the diet, antiflatulents, metoclopramide, domperidone, or chlorpromazine. In the chest, intractable cough and dyspnoea may occur owing to obstructive airways disease or inadequate chest-wall movement, or because of the intrusions of pneumonia or cardiac failure. The appropriate treatment might include steroids for bronchospasm, diuretics and oxygen for cardiac failure, or morphine to control respiratory distress in appropriate circumstances.

Restlessness, confusion, and insomnia are common accompaniments of the aging brain, often initiated by anoxia, infections, pain, and minor injuries; they respond well to small doses of chloral or promazine, but if they are caused by pain, analgesics must be given. Pruritus can be intractable, especially if due to jaundice or malignancy; some relief may be obtained by cholestyramine or anabolic steroids, or occasionally by antihistamines, whose sedative effects may be beneficial in the terminal state. Aspirin, codeine, NSAIDs, steroids, morphine, or local nerve blocks may be necessary to overthrow the symptoms of metastatic bone pain.

There is no obligation on the physician to prolong life at all costs; the prevention and relief of distress should be his ever-conscious aim. Doctors of a bygone era were probably more adept in this than the technologically-obsessed modern generation. A physician's duty should not end with a referral to a hospice; they are of varied quality and expertise. Time spent with the sufferer and his family, and frank but informal discussions of the patient's apprehensions—including death itself—can be confronted with much advantage.

Sir William Jenner commended the qualities he considered essential to a medical man: 'He needs three things. He must be honest, he must be dogmatic, and he must be kind.' In imparting good counsel to the terminal patient, physicians need all these attributes, but perhaps the last above the rest.

Osler's insistence on *aequanimitas* and a cheerful optimism is a valuable weapon in the face of death and dying. 'It is the hardest stone one can throw a man to remove all hope' said Gavey in his humane and penetrating essay;[4] we should always be able to find words of encouragement and measured optimism.

With suitable and attentive medical and nursing care and a frank and open relationship with families, most patients can die in peace and dignity, freed from pain and distress.

References

1. Scott, S., Caird, F. I., and Williams, B. O. (1985). Communication in Parkinson's disease. Croom Helm, London.
2. Anonymous. (1990). Leading article: driving and Parkinson's disease. *Lancet*, **336**, 781.
3. Hindmarch, I. and Gudgeon, A. C. (1980). The effects of clobazam and lorazepam on aspects of psychomotor performance and car driving ability. *British Journal of Clinical Pharmacology* **10**, 145–50.
4. Gavey, C. J. (1952). The management of the 'hopeless case'. Buckston Browne Prize Essay, Harveian Society of London, 1950. H.K. Lewis, London.

15 Conclusions

Parkinson's disease remains something of an enigma. The main problem is a lack of dopamine, which as we have seen can be effectively replaced by modern drug treatment. This permits a full and active life for many years in most subjects. The Parkinson's Disease Society and other organizations fund medical and social research on a very large scale. As a result, hardly a year goes by without some important addition to knowledge—additions which are of practical importance to each and every sufferer from the disease. But all such discoveries require careful scientific scrutiny before they can be accepted as valid.

The present excitement about nigral transplants is a good example. But, for the moment, no victim of Parkinson's disease should feel in any way deprived of this unproven procedure. Indeed, the early euphoric responses to the notion of adrenal transplants have been dashed on the rocks of clinical experience. The benefits of fetal nigral transplants are presently tentative speculations based on small numbers of patients who have experienced different experimental and surgical approaches. But transplants are being tested in the UK and Scandinavia, and if they are proved to be worthwhile will be applied sensibly in due course.

Future prospects

The main aims of research must be to pursue the essential cause or causes of the syndrome and to prevent the onset of illness. This may mean identifying individuals at risk before the first symptoms emerge, or preferably earlier still, for the disease is almost certainly of many years duration before the advent of symptoms. An alternative but complementary prospect is the identification of preclinical disease. If this is achieved, some form of protective therapy may be feasible. We know, for example, that preclinical detection of dopaminergic damage can now be demonstrated by diminished 6-fluorodopa uptake in the striatum on PET scanning in asymptomatic patients with exposure to MPTP—an acute brain insult. The assumption is that there is a prolonged period of dopamine depletion in idiopathic disease, and this is supported by the singular finding of Lewy bodies in a sympathectomy specimen removed for hypertension years before Parkinson's disease became manifest. But PET scanning is unlikely to be a practical screening method for many years, and we lack other valid predictors of disease.

One suggestion is that certain neuropsychological defects are present before the emergence of physical symptoms and signs. Constructional tasks, category naming, the Rosen drawing test, and the Stroop word colour test have been found to be abnormal in non-demented parkinsonian subjects and in relatively asymptomatic MPTP-exposed subjects with abnormal PET scans. It is unlikely, however, that these relatively selective cognitive abnormalities will be specific for pre-symptomatic dopamine depletion, since the abnormalities are probably of high sensitivity but of low specificity.

Other suggestions have been the search for the well documented but often asymptomatic hyposmia or anosmia seen in Parkinson's disease irrespective of the severity and duration of the motor syndrome. The idea of applying tests of smell as a screening method is attractive for its simplicity; but it too is certain to be of low specificity. The detection of abnormal and prolonged visual evoked potentials (VEPs) has also been demonstrated in variable numbers of patients, but would seem likely to be insensitive and again non-specific.

Biological markers have been mentioned in Chapter 6, and attempts have been made to utilize several of these as preclinical detectors. Sadly, however, abnormalities are common in motor-neurone disease, Alzheimer's disease, and other neurodegenerative disorders. Mito-chondrial Complex-1 presents the most exciting area of research at the moment, but plainly brain material is inaccessible. The depletion of Complex-1 in platelets is a possible line for future investigation. Abnormalities in the metabolic handling of debrisoquine, acetamino-phen, and S-carboxymethyl-L-cysteine have been described as other possible biochemical markers. There remain considerable technical problems in the widespread application of these methods, and their specificity is in doubt. It is possible that combinations of a battery of tests might be a more accurate method of preclinical detection, but, as is so often the case, we are obliged to conclude that although the direction and purpose of future investigation is well signposted, much further research is needed.

There are many other avenues of progress under investigation. Although we are dealing with a slowly progressing illness in most cases, patients should remember that most victims have a near-normal lifespan, which includes many years of activity and enjoyment. Sufferers from Parkinson's disease can face the future with measured optimism.

Appendix: Information, publications, and benefits for Parkinson's disease patients and families

Support groups

Parkinson's Disease Society, 36 Portland Place, London W1N 3DG. Tel: 071-255 2432.

Young Alert Parkinson's Partners and Relatives (YAPP&RS), The Yapper, 6 King's Meadow, King's Langley, Herts WD4 8RT.

Publications and information

Stern, G. and Lees, A. (1990). *Parkinson's disease: the facts*, (2nd edn). Oxford University Press.

Help for handicapped people. A DSS booklet available from the Parkinson's Disease Society or your local Social Security office.

Disability rights handbook. Available from The Disability Alliance, 25 Denmark Street, London WC2 8NJ. Price £4.00, post free.

Coping with disablement. Published by the Consumers Association, 14 Buckingham Street, London WC2N 6DS.

Holidays for the physically handicapped. Available from the Central Council for the Disabled, 34 Ecclestone Square, London SW1V 1PE.

Disabled Living Foundation, 346 Kensington High Street, London W14 8NS. Advice about equipment and aids.

Citizen's Advice Bureau, local information. See local telephone directory.

Benefits

A number of benefits are available to selected patients depending on their clinical condition, disabilities, and in some instances a medical report. Not every patient is entitled to all benefits. Specific sums quoted are correct at the time of writing but will be subject to alterations.

1. Orange car badge, the Disabled badge, permits parking concessions and freedom from some tolls; apply to local council offices. Remember that when you have Parkinsons' disease you are required to notify the DVLC, Swansea, who will allow a driving licence if the disability is not considered to be dangerous.

2. Mobility allowance, tax-free, £26.55/week; also entitles one to orange badge and possible exemption from road tax. Walking distance must be very restricted. Apply for leaflet N1211 from the DSS.

3. Invalidity Benefit, tax-free. This is payable after 28 weeks of claiming sickness benefit. It is £46.90/week, paid up to the age of 70. Obtain form SSP1 from employer after 22 weeks' statutory sick pay.

4. Attendance allowance, tax-free. If you can demonstrate the need for care, whether or not you live alone. £25.05/week for day-care alone; £37.55/week when night- and day-care are necessary. Obtain leaflet N1205 from the DSS.

5. Invalid Care allowance. Payable to the carer in certain conditions. £28.20/week, plus additions in certain circumstances. Obtain leaflet N1212 from the DSS.

6. Free prescriptions under certain conditions, for example, if you are unable to leave home alone. Obtain leaflet P11 from the DSS or a post office.

Index